Power & Politics in Nursing Administration:

A CASEBOOK

Power & Politics in Nursing Administration:

A CASEBOOK

Dorothy J. del Bueno, Ed.D., R.N.
Cynthia M. Freund, Ph.D., R.N.

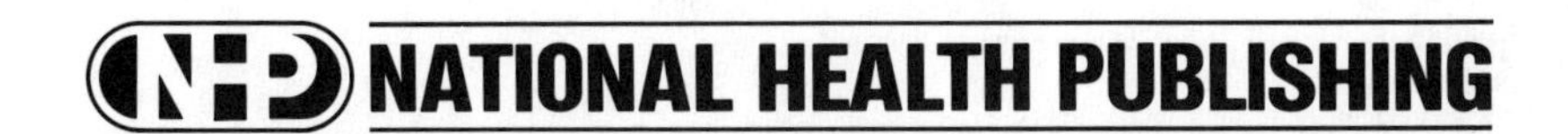

99 Painters Mill Road
Owings Mills, MD 21117

Printed in the United States of America
First Printing
ISBN: 0-932500-42-0
LC: 86-60385

Contents

PART III **Analysis of Selected Cases**

PART IV **Readings on Power and Politics in Organizations**

Foreword

Today's nurse administrator must, above all, be creative: not the left-brain-logic, right-brain-artistic dichotomous creativity as defined in yesteryear. Today's nurse administrator needs the type of creativity defined by Emily Smith in a *Business Week* cover story on creativity. Smith says that recent research is defining creativity as a feat of mental gymnastics engaging the conscious and subconscious parts of the brain, drawing on knowledge, logic, imagination, intuition, and the ability to make the connections and distinctions between ideas and things. This type of creativity is essential for good problem-solving (including finding the right question, not just the right answer), dealing with change (or deciding when not to), and meeting diverse people needs while getting a product "out the door." All of this must be done using techniques congruent with a unique organizational culture.

In addition to creativity, today's nursing administrator must have a vision. This leader needs to be focused, share a dream, articulate simple, shared values, and bring the followers along as a team. Dedication, futuristic goal orientation, a real concern for colleagues, and astute awareness (from both the formal and informal systems) are apparent in the visionary nursing administrator.

The creative nurse administrator with a vision needs one more basic ingredient--the ability to get a product "out the door." Since the mid-1970s recession, this cold hard fact has resurfaced to haunt, and even destroy, many executives and their companies. The health care industry companies have been no exception. In fact, this industry, formerly third-party-payment sheltered from the close scrutiny and responsibility for health care funds, felt the mid-1970s and subsequent financial constraints more than most industries . . . and were most unprepared to handle business from this financially accountable position.

Being creative, sharing a vision, and maintaining high productivity all need to be done within the reality of a particular organization's culture. These are the pieces, beyond task and people responsibilities, that *make* today's nursing executive a success--these are the sources of your power and the basis of your politics within your organization. How does all this work? Dorothy del Bueno and Cynthia Freund provide vital clues to help you realize your creativity, vision, and productivity goals within the reality of your complex bureaucratic political setting. The authors share realistic experiences through case studies that make you say "ah ha" on a subject of power and politics that is most often learned by falling into each pitfall. They offer clear analyses of selected cases to help you "learn from others." And, the authors present a model for politically astute planning and decision-making to keep you on the right track. *Power and Politics in Nursing Administration* is a must for nursing administration executives--unless you have the time and energy in your career to learn by falling into the pitfalls.

Duane Walker, M.S., R.N., F.A.A.N.
Vice President, Queens Medical Center
Honolulu, Hawaii

Special Acknowledgments

A special acknowledgment is given to the individuals who were willing to share their stories with the authors and who provided us with additional insights into the effect power, politics, and personality all have on ultimate success as a nursing service administrator.

We would also like to thank Kleia R. Luckner, CNM, of the Northwest Ohio Center for Women and Children, who assisted with the development of the organizational culture checklist. Her ideas and suggestions were extremely helpful.

And last, but not least, the authors gratefully acknowledge the first group of graduate students in the Kellogg Administration Program, School of Nursing, University of Pennsylvania, who provided considerable assistance and valuable insight to the case study analyses. Many thanks to Carin Carlson, Judith Ann Jones, Virginia Maroun, Steven Rabinowitz, and Charlotte Santoferro.

Dorothy J. del Bueno
Cynthia M. Freund

About the Authors

Dorothy Joan del Bueno, Ed.D., R.N., is Assistant Dean for Continuing Education and Acting Director of the Kellogg Administration Program at the University of Pennsylvania. In addition to her bachelor's and doctorate from Columbia University, she holds a master's degree in nursing from New York University. Her professional experience includes positions in both in-service nursing and nursing administration and education. More than 60 of her articles have appeared in the major nursing journals, and she is presently a member of the advisory board for the *Journal of Nursing Administration.* Since 1972 she has traveled extensively across the country giving workshops in nursing personnel management and developing educational programs and performance appraisal systems for a wide range of health care institutions. From 1978 to 1980 she served as Chairperson for the Council on Continuing Education of the American Nurses' Association.

Cynthia M. Freund, Ph.D., R.N., is Associate Professor of Nursing at the University of North Carolina at Chapel Hill. Her bachelor's and master's degrees in nursing are from Marquette University and the University of North Carolina, respectively, and she holds the doctorate in administration from the University of Alabama. A certified family nurse practitioner, she has held various in-service, academic, research, and consulting positions and is the author of a number of publications in nursing administration and on the nurse practitioner profession. In 1977-1978 she served as Vice-Chairperson on the Council of Family Nurse Practitioners and Clinicians of the American Nurses' Association.

About the Authors

How to Use This Book

It is always easy to be wise and objective when not directly involved in a problem situation or event. It is also true that hindsight is more reliable than foresight or conjecture. All of the cases in this book represent very complex organizational problems that could be perceived and understood from many perspectives. Bolman and Deal (1984) have described and defined four perspectives or frames that they believe represent the major schools of organizational thought. They have labeled these perspectives or frames the structural, the human resource, the political, and the symbolic.

The structural frame emphasizes the importance of formal roles and relationships. Structures are created to fit an organization's environment and technology. The human resource frame bases its beliefs on peoples' needs, feelings, and prejudices. People make up organizations; therefore the key to effectiveness is to tailor the organization to fit the people. The political frame views organizations as arenas of scarce resources where power and influence determine the allocation of the resources. Conflict is expected. Bargaining, coercion, and coalition-forming are a way of life. The symbolic frame focuses on irrationality and describes the organization as a theatre or carnival.

Organizations are held together by shared values and culture rather than by goals and policies (Bolman and Deal 1984, pp. 4-6). Each frame has a vision of reality that may be incompatible with another view. Each frame has the tendency to predict, describe, or explain what happens in organizations based on a self-fulfilling prophecy approach. We find what we look for.

The authors of this book have purposefully chosen to emphasize two of the four frames described. Although there are elements of the structural and human resource frames identified in the case studies, the primary focus is the political and the symbolic. "The political perspective is an important antidote to the antiseptic rationality that sometimes characterizes rational perspective and naive optimism present in human resource theories . . . The political frame results in two major implications for action: (1) those who increase their power and their political sophistication win more battles than they lose; (2) most efforts to make organizations more rational or humane are likely to fail," (Bolman and Deal 1984, p. 216).

The political perspective views organizations as coalitions of individuals and interest groups who have different objectives and resources, with each individual or interest group attempting to influence the goals and decisions of the organization. The political perspective acknowledges the importance of group needs, but focuses on scarce resources and incompatible demands when different interests are in conflict. Such conflicts are a fact of life to be dealt with to the advantage of some and to the disadvantage of others. From a political perspective, conflict is not a negative, but something natural and inevitable. Power from any source--authority, expertise, personality, control of resources, or association with powerful others--is a priority commodity to be effectively wheeled and dealed. In the political perspective, players come and go. Today's winners are tomorrow's losers, but the game goes on. Significant change occurs only when there are significant shifts in the balance of power.

The symbolic perspective emphasizes that what is most important about any event is the meaning of what happened to those involved. "Symbols serve three major functions in organizations: (a) economy, (b) elaboration to resolve ambiguity and give meaning, and (c) valuation and prophecy suggesting how to feel and how to evaluate events. Symbols provide purpose, faith, and positive myth. Many organizational phenomena that appear dysfunctional when viewed in the light of their ostensible purposes, are logical and predictable in view of their symbolic functions.'' (Bolman and Deal 1984, p. 218). The symbolic frame assumes that organizations have many questions and problems that have no real answers or solutions. People use symbols to manage the chaos, confusion, and unpredictability of these situations. Symbols most frequently used are myths, rituals, ceremonies, stories, and humor.

Each perspective or frame has advantages and disadvantages. Bolman and Deal believe that the symbolic and political perspectives are most useful when resources are declining or scarce, change is rapid, uncertainty is high, and organizations are older. These characteristics are descriptive of many health care organizations, particularly hospitals. Professional schools, in preparing graduates for their technical specialty such as nursing, medicine, or law, do little to prepare their graduates for the idiosyncrasies of organizational life. Professional school graduates ''know very little about organizational and political culture; hence, they are quite unsure about what questions to ask, what work habits are considered acceptable, who to get to know, how much to talk and what to talk about'' (Raelin 1985, p. 153). Many professionals are naive in their belief that organizational success rests on their demonstrated technical expertise and competence (Raelin 1985, p. 153).

There is a critical change at some point in the management hierarchy when the key to success shifts toward influencing the organization as a whole, not just the subordinate group. This point, referred to as breakpoint leadership, places a heavy emphasis on political and diplomatic skills and requires the exercise of power without guilt. Breakpoint leadership requires knowing how the organization works, what are its cultural norms, and how to use power and influence to get things done (Hill and Collins-Eaglin 1985, p. 186). For these reasons the authors have chosen to present the case studies within the context of the political and symbolic frames. We have purposefully chosen to report cases that are reflective of power, politics, and culture, variables believed to be particularly relevant to managerial success and failure in health care organizations. We can never be sure of course, if our presentation, representation, and interpretation of the reported facts and events are totally valid. However, we hope these cases will shed some light on very real, very common situations. By so doing we hope present and future nursing service administrators who find themselves in similar situations will be helped to manage such situations effectively and successfully.

PART I

A Conceptual Framework for Success in Organizations

Power and Politics in Organizations

Political realists see the world as it is: an arena of power politics moved primarily by perceived immediate self interests, where morality is rhetorical rationale for expedient action and self interest. It is a world not of angels but of angles, where men speak of moral principles but act as power principles; a world where we are always moral and our enemies always immoral.

Saul Alinsky, *Rules for Radicals*, pp. 12-13

Why do some managers and executives fail, some succeed, and some just keep running in place? What is the secret for success in organizations? The contemporary nurse executive, to be successful and effective, must have "expertise that extends beyond the planning, controlling, and other classical managerial functions" (Ehrat 1983, p. 29). By the time a manager reaches a certain level or rank in an organization, success and failure have little to do with performance or accomplishments, but a great deal to do with "social factors, determined by authority and political alignments . . . and the ethics and style of the organization" (Jackall 1983, p. 122). Performance is always subject to a myriad of interpretations, almost always within the context of the norms and values of the organization. "Managers are the quintessential bureaucratic work group; they not only fashion bureaucratic rules, they are also bound by them. Managers are not just in the organization, they are of the organization" (Jackall 1983, p. 119). Organizations themselves

FIGURE 1

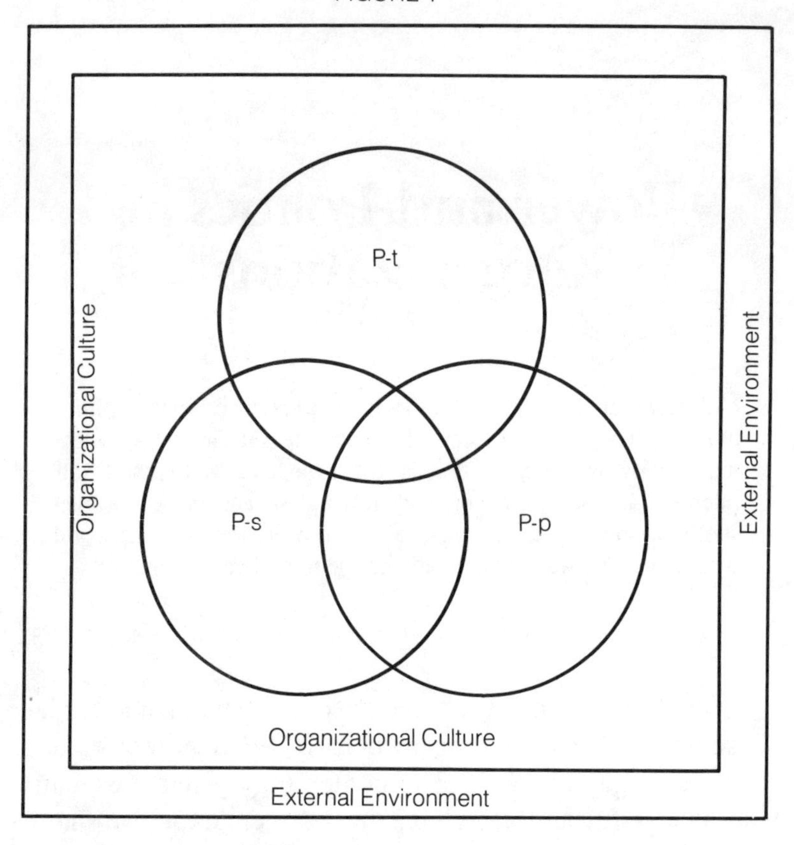

do not exist in a vacuum, but are part of a larger context or environment.

This concept of managers and executives exercising a variety of skills and behaviors within an organizational culture and external environment is graphically illustrated in Figure 1. The three equal, overlapping circles represent the three major dimensions of skills and abilities required of successful managers and executives. *P-t* represents performance of technical skills such as planning, delegating, and problem solving. *P-s* represents managerial style or the use of interpersonal skills and self to relate to individuals and groups. *P-p* represents the political skills needed to obtain and keep power. Although these three circles are shown as equal in size, they may not be equal in importance. The size of the circles and the relationship among them will depend upon the inner square representing the organization's culture or norms. This inner square is set within an outer square labeled external environment. The effective, successful manager or executive will be knowledgeable about all of these elements and understand the relationships among and between the parts. Most classic management texts, with the exception of Machiavelli's *The Prince*, emphasize and describe only technical performance requirements (P-t) or managerial style (P-s). Recently the phenomena of organizational culture and politics have been acknowledged as an important component in organizational success. This chapter describes the nature and importance of the acquisition and use of political skills. The chapter that follows focuses on organizational culture and norms as another important component for success within an organization.

Power and Political Know-How

"The most important and unyielding necessity of organizational life is not better communication, human relations, or employee participation, but power--or the capacity to modify the conduct of others while avoiding modification of one's own behavior. Power is acquired, not given, and essentially is held by political means" (McMurray 1973, p. 69). Friedrich Nietzsche, Arthur Schopenhauer, and Alfred Adler all believed that the power motive is the most fundamental urge in human nature. All three also believed that politics and the pursuit of status within hierarchies motivate a great percentage of human behavior in organizations. Bertrand Russell, another philosopher, has been credited with saying that much that passes as idealism is a disguised love of power,

"Ambivalent attitudes toward power and its use, together with the lack of useful information about power in management, breed both naive and cynical beliefs about what effective and successful managers do'' (Kotter 1979, p. 5). The same can be said about politics, another avoided or ''dirty'' word. There is nothing inherently good or evil about power or politics. Power is the ability to get another person to behave in a way contrary to his or her immediate or long-range interests. It is how, when, and by whom power is used that will determine desirable or undesirable outcomes and short- and long-term effects. ''To become a sophisticated organizational member requires the development of skills to cope with the facts of power without being forced into submissiveness against one's will . . . '' (Randsepp 1984, p. 40). It is vital to have a realistic view of how organizations actually operate in order to forestall victimization by the inevitable power politics of the system.

Organizations are made up of people who are constantly vying with one another for power, status, and prestige. A certain amount of politics is therefore inevitable, since everyone, or almost everyone, wants to increase his or her share of these three elements that are important for organizational success. ''Organizations' political systems are reflected in who gets ahead, how they get rewarded, and who has power to make what decisions'' (Tichy 1983, p. 45). An individual is perceived and acknowledged as powerful or influential by others when that person uses political savvy, has an obvious power base and network, and has more than a fair share of scarce resources. ''Three commodities are necessary for accumulating productive power--information, resources and support'' (Kanter 1982, p. 98). ''The primary reason power dynamics emerge and play an important role in organizations is not necessarily because managers are power hungry, or because they want desperately to get ahead, or even because there is an inherent conflict between managers who have authority and workers who do not. Power is important because the dependence inherent in managerial jobs is greater than the power or control given to the people in those jobs'' (Kotter 1979, p. 16). Successful managers therefore need to go beyond the limits of their formal positions. For this they need power.

Power bases are those resources available to an individual that give the person the ability to convince others to go along. Few power bases are given; they must be grasped, taken, cajoled, or impounded. Power bases, political strategies, and the art of deception may seem far removed from the direct task of problem diagnosis and solution intervention. Failure to develop tactical skills and political savvy, however, is unrealistic and may even be harmful to an executive's organizational success. Maintaining one's place in the organization is known as power politics--the human equivalent to pecking order in the animal world.

Power plays, or political struggles, are often reflected in the allocation of scarce resources. In times of economic scarcity, political activity increases as individuals compete for those declining resources. A power holder must not only have control of valued resources, but must be willing to use them to influence others. To produce results, power, like money, needs to circulate. When power is hoarded it atrophies and blocks achievement. In reality, organizations operate in a way similar to the working of the political arena where everyone is jockeying for power and influence. Managers use both offensive and defensive techniques to acquire and maintain the power necessary to function and achieve their objectives.

Machiavelli's advice, to be both a lion and a fox--to know when to use force and when to use cunning--appears still to have relevance for life in today's organizations. His fine Italian hand would seem to be behind memos that distort or omit information, meetings held to decide that which has already been decided, coalitions formed to block a decision, and rewards promised but never received (Schein 1985, p. 1).

Political Strategies and Tactics

Political strategies for getting or keeping power include coalition forming, bargaining or trade-offs, lobbying, posturing or bluffing, and increasing visibility. Coalition forming is the temporary joining of individuals with a common purpose or goal in order to increase the individual's ability to bring pressure on superiors or peers in another department.

Bargaining, or trade-offs, requires that each side or participant has something the other wants and also something they are willing to give up. Some of the things that can be traded are concrete, such as space or personnel, whereas others are abstractions, such as support and ideas. Whatever the trade-offs, they should be relatively equal in order to avoid one participant or party ending up being in debt to the other participant.

Posturing or bluffing is a major bargaining tactic in which more is asked than is ever expected and in which fallback positions are always possible. Posturing is an attempt to keep others off balance or to keep them guessing about what is really wanted.

Increasing visibility is a strategy in which an individual consciously engages in activities that lead to being in the right place at the right time with the right people. Such activities may include participation in committees, on task forces, at social gatherings, or on special projects. These activities will obviously be related to pet projects, vested interests, or hidden agendas of important or powerful individuals.

One of the positive aspects of using politics is that it can help cut through bureaucratic red tape. How political a manager or executive should be obviously depends on the organization's values and norms in relation to politicizing and power brokering. If used exclusively or incongruently with organizational norms, politicizing may backfire or cause distrust. "As a general rule, it is those who are or who become politically vulnerable or expendable who get set up and become blamable . . . diffusion of responsibility inevitably means that someone, somewhere is going to become a scapegoat when things go wrong" (Jackall 1983, p. 126). Thus it is obvious that successful managers and executives must make intelligent, creative, and purposeful use of political strategies. "Power struggles, alliance formation, strategic maneuvering, and cutthroat actions

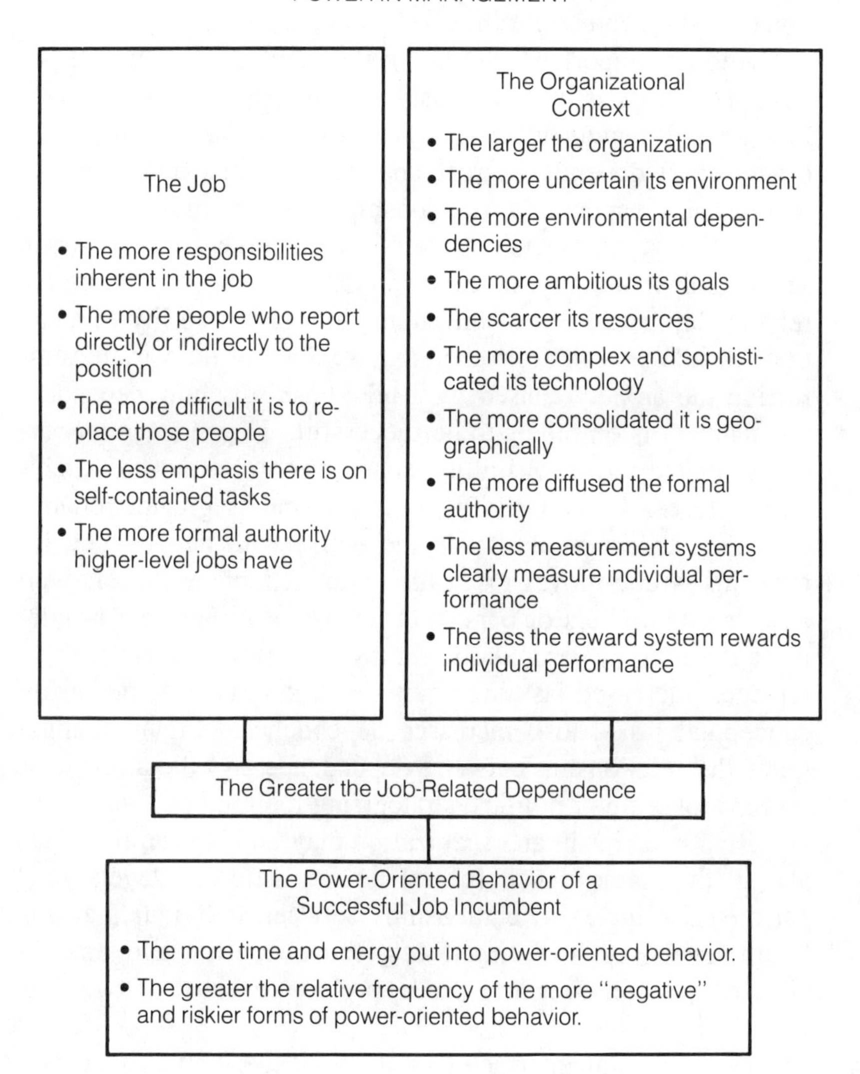

Figure 2. Relationship between the power-oriented behavior of an effective manager and key situational contingencies.

may be as endemic to organizational life as planning, organizing, directing, and controlling'' (Schein, p. 1).

Another important variable in the success or failure of political strategies is the relationships managers recognize, establish, and ultimately manage. The effective functioning of an organization depends a great deal on the ebbs and flows of feelings and responses to relationships between individuals and groups. Two key variables interact and influence behavior in relationships: anxiety, or the response to stress imposed by the relationship, and level of differentiation, or the ability to adapt to or detach oneself from the anxiety. One of the variables affecting the anxiety caused by a relationship is how dependent the manager is on others to be successful. Dependence on others is related to responsibility, span of control, and task ambiguity. Greater responsibility usually requires greater reliance on others to cooperate or do the work, with dependency increasing as one moves up in the organization. Managers who have large numbers of personnel reporting to them are usually more dependent, particularly if those reporting are difficult to replace. Increased task ambiguity, or a job that includes many conceptual tasks, also increases dependence. Figure 2 illustrates the relationship between dependence and the amount of power brokering or political strategizing required of a manager.

Relationships in an organization may be between individuals at the same level (peers) or at different levels (superior/subordinate). Relationships between individuals at different levels, or level interfaces, cause conflict and anxiety when they differ over an issue or problem because of overt inequality in power.

Departmental interfaces, or relationships between departments exist when subunits of an organization are interdependent on one another to accomplish their objectives or goals and therefore must interact. An example is the interface between the pharmacy and nursing departments of a hospital. Even though these departments do not have a formal authority or reporting relationship, they may have unequal power in the organization. Thus conflict and anxiety are common in departmental interface relationships.

Relationships between individuals or groups with different, incompatible, or conflicting values and norms are called cultural interfaces. Cultural interfaces or relationships can exist between different age groups, between groups or individuals of different sex, between different religious affiliations or ethnic backgrounds, or a combination of any of these. Cultural interfaces between doctors and nurses usually involve age, gender, and social background differences. A high level of anxiety often results from overt and covert power differences across cultural interfaces.

Many of the most problematic conflicts in organizations involve individuals acting for groups. In these instances it is difficult for individuals to separate self-interests and personal values from the group's best interests or needs. Since under conditions of threat people usually act competitively to protect themselves, even at the expense of the group or the organization, a great deal of anxiety can be generated in this kind of interface or relationship. Resolving such conflicts requires considerable managerial skill.

Some of these skills and tactics are described on the following pages. Not all may be acceptable to all nurse executives, but they do have high probability of success.

• ***Build your own team.*** Many executives have discovered too late their vulnerability to sabotage by disgruntled, disappointed, or jealous subordinates inherited from another manager. New managers are particularly at risk when coming in from the outside because of not knowing "where the bodies are buried" (McMurray 1973, p. 70).

• ***Choose your second-in-command carefully.*** "An aggressive, ambitious, upwardly mobile number two man (or woman) is dangerous and often difficult to control" (McMurray 1973, p. 70).

• ***Establish alliances with both superiors and peers.*** This is done by determining the other person's expectations and motivations. Choose your friends carefully, however. It may be necessary to form alliances with many who will not be true friends. True friends are those to whom you can bare your soul and whom you can rely upon in a conflict of interest.

• ***Use all possible channels of communication***. Deal and Kennedy (1982, p. 92-94) identify the roles of spies and whisperers, or individuals who will bring and spread information. Without both upward and downward channels of communication, the executive becomes isolated and subject to being preempted or ousted in power struggles.

• ***Know when to be fair to subordinates.*** Being fair to aggressive, manipulative people is tantamount to letting them take over one's power and perhaps even one's job.

• ***Don't be naive about how decisions are made.*** Ideas and changes rarely stand on their own merit. Awareness of the pervasive influence of powerful people and their biases is crucial to predicting how a decision will be made.

• ***Know what takes priority.*** A vice-president of a Boston consulting firm, describes three kinds of routines people perform in organizations. The first are task routines, or those things performed simply to get the job done. The second set of routines consists of survival tasks, or those things done to protect self and position. The third set are camouflage routines, or those things done to disguise the use of survival routines.

• ***Be courteous.*** Courtesy is one of the most effective power tools. Courtesy makes others feel good or powerful and keeps them from feeling put-down--a perception that is sure to lead to retaliation or power politics. Executives whose power needs are satisfied are usually courteous to others, particularly to those in subordinate positions.

• ***Maintain a flexible position and maneuverability.*** Commit yourself to only a few uncompromisable positions on issues that are ethically or morally essential to you. Maneuverability allows for graceful adaptation to changing circumstances or power bases. In line with this strategy is willingness to compromise on small issues. Don't confuse trivia with the main events.

• ***Use deception judiciously.*** Schein (1985, p. 4) describes two types of organizational climates, dynamic and static, and two different motivations, personal and organizational. Personal motives include career advancement, status, money, and recognition. Such intents are not necessarily related to organizational goals such as profit, image, market share, and customer satisfaction. Static systems are those that require a minimum level of productive energy to maintain viability in a relatively stable environment. Dynamic organizations are those operating in a highly competitive environment and therefore requiring rapid and nonroutine decision making accompanied by high-energy output. In dynamic organizations, managers focus more on organization goals than on personal motivations. The opposite is true in static organizations. In static organizations managers often engage in political warfare to satisfy their need for excitement and challenge. "Deception and intrigue add interest to the otherwise routine and even-keel environment . . . Political warfare, by revving up the system, fosters the illusion that it is active, filled with excitement and competition. The reality of a perhaps boring system need never be faced. Thus, deception and illusion keep members involved in the organization and provide needed rewards" (Schein 1985, p. 4). Even in dynamic organizations it may be necessary to practice some deception in regard to how one uses the power strategies--trading, coalition forming, and contacts--in order to operate effectively (Schein 1985, p. 4).

• ***Use passive resistance*** when under pressure from demands that you cannot openly challenge or that are not in your best interest. Stall or take steps that delay real action toward the undesired goal or objective.

• ***Project an image of status, power, and material success.*** "Most people measure a leader by the degree of pomp and circumstance surrounding him. This is why the king lives in a palace and the Pope in the Vatican. Too much modesty and democracy may easily be mistaken for lack of power and influence" (McMurray 1973, p. 74).

• ***Learn to "swim with sharks."*** Assume that strangers or unknowns are the enemy or competitors until you have evidence to the contrary. Counter any aggression promptly with obvious retaliation. Do not be ingratiating or conciliatory. Even better, anticipate aggression and move first. Take your adversary by surprise. Divert an organized attack by initiating internal dissension. Introduce an issue or rumor that sets your adversaries to fighting among themselves. And above all, don't "bleed," at least not in public (Cousteau 1978).

Conclusion

Despite the abstract nature of the concept of power, it is a variable of any work setting. Because it is part of reality, it must be accepted, understood, and used. Too frequently women make the mistake of trying to rise above power plays and politics, only to find themselves left out of important decisions. Used wisely, constructively, and judiciously, power promotes achievement of goals and objectives (Chater 1983, p. 334). Power and its potential abuses can be controlled by accepting and understanding its nature and use. "The position of an executive is often perilous with little inherent security. If things go well, tenure in the position is secure; if things go badly, the executive may be made the scapegoat . . . the only hope for survival under conditions over which the executive may have little or no control, is to gain power by tactics that are in a large measure political, and by means that are, in part at least, Machiavellian. Such strategies and tactics are not always noble and high-minded. But neither are they naive. Rather, they have one primary merit: they enhance chances of survival" (McMurray, p. 74).

Organizational Culture

Every organization, like every community, has cultural norms and values. In some organizations these norms and values are overt and pervasive, while in others they may be subtle and difficult to discern. Culture, another word for social reality, is both product and process. It is the shaper of human interaction and of the outcomes generated by ongoing interactions (Jelinek 1982, p. 331). Culture gives meaning to the myriad of behaviors and practices recognized as a distinct way of life in communities, special interest groups, and organizations. Because norms and values are an integral part of decisions made related to what we do, say, and feel, culture has a powerful effect on behavior.

"Whether one treats the culture as a background factor, an organizational variable, or as a metaphor for conceptualization, the idea of culture focuses attention on the expressive, nonrational qualities of the organization and legitimates attention to its subjective, interpretive aspects" (Smircich 1983, p. 355). Successful managers both recognize cultural indicators and make conscious decisions about compliance or noncompliance with the norms and values of the culture.

Importance of Organizational Culture

Suddenly everyone is talking and writing about organizational culture. Culture is in. What has precipitated this current interest in the phenomenon or reality of organizational culture?

Wilkins (1983) suggests that recent turbulence in the United STates economy has accelerated the need for organizations to look within themselves and analyze the reasons for their success or failure. Strong company cultures can either motivate coordinated action to achieve needed innovation or can serve as strong barriers to required changes such as diversification, downsizing, retrenchment, or reorganization (Wilkins 1983, p. 24-25). In organizations, such as hospitals, that are undergoing rapid and stressful changes it will be important not only to understand the existing culture but also to identify the need and means to redirect the culture.

On an individual level, cultural understanding is necessary for people to function in a given setting. Employees need a continuing sense of the reality of what the setting is all about. Culture is the system of such publicly and collectively accepted meaning. Culture fills the gap between the formal language of the employment contract and the way things work in the real world (Pettigrew 1979, p. 570). Organizational norms often become apparent to employees when they change roles, when they are promoted, or when their job function is altered. Novices and newcomers often unknowingly violate taken-for-granted norms related to the way the job is to be done or the way relationships are established. The offending newcomer may be shunned, ridiculed, lectured, or given friendly advice about his *faux pas*. When the offending individual finally gets the real message, he or she is rewarded, accepted, and treated like everyone else.

Every organization has a culture composed of shared beliefs and values, a kind of normative glue that holds the organization together. ''Whether weak or strong, culture has a powerful influence throughout an organization; it affects practically everything--from who gets promoted and what decisions are made, to how employees dress and what sports they play,'' (Deal and Kennedy 1982, p. 4).

''In any given organization and situation, there are limits or boundaries of tolerance beyond which behavior, decisions, or actions will not be accepted, and beyond which consequences will follow'' (Ehrat 1983, p. 32). These limits are more or less clearly defined. The values and beliefs of the organizational culture determine what matters are to be attended to, what kind of information is to be taken most seriously, and what kind of people are most respected. Organizations that have strong cultures maintain those cultures by managing their human resources: who is let into the organization, how they are developed, and how they are rewarded. The challenge for successful managers is to understand the organizational culture well enough to be able to tailor their behavior and strategies to comply with existing norms and values. For example, if the norm requires that everyone be consulted on all problems, it is important that a manager gets everyone's advice before announcing or proposing a managerial decision. Many managers and executives fail, not because of incompetence or poor performance, but because they do not acknowledge or correctly interpret the organizational culture.

Definitions of Organizational Culture

Organizational culture, like any other culture, is the taken-for-granted and shared meaning that members of the culture assign to their social surroundings and subsequently reinforce. The key to understanding a culture lies in how the members of the culture structure the meaning of their world.

``Culture, conceived as shared key values and beliefs, fulfills several important functions. First, it conveys a sense of identity for organization members. Second, it facilitates the generation of commitment to something larger than self. Third, it enhances social system stability, and fourth, it serves as a sense-making device that guides and shapes behavior'' (Smircich 1983, p. 346).

Culture, as a metaphor for organizations, allows us to go beyond the mechanical or instrumental view of organizations. Organizations cannot be understood in economic terms only, but must be considered in relation to their symbolic and expressive aspects.

The importance of accurate symbolic interpretation is related to a set of basic assumptions about the nature of both organizations and human beings (Bolman and Deal 1984). These assumptions include the following:

- What is most important about an event is the meaning or interpretation given to it.
- Many significant events are unclear or ambiguous in their meaning and therefore need interpretation.
- When faced with uncertainty or ambiguity, people create symbols to reduce confusion and provide a logical explanation.

"Symbolism assumes that organizations are full of questions that cannot be answered, problems that cannot be solved, and events that cannot be understood or managed (Bolman and Deal 1984, p. 152). Culture is the total of the symbols, language, and behaviors that make up the organization's norms and values.

A number of metaphors and analogies are used to describe organizational culture: military, sports, anthropological, and mechanistic, to name a few. Figures of speech, or tropes are illustrative of the metaphor used. Consider the following: "This place is a jungle," "This place is a battlefield," "We run a tight ship here," "We are one big happy family," "We function like a well-oiled machine," "The XYZ department is the heart of this organization." Such language is a clue to the organization's self-perception of its cultural orientation.

It is important, of course, to look both for consistency in the symbolic language and for the meaning behind the symbols. Meaning is rarely spoken of openly, but is inferred from what people say and do. Stories and rituals often are helpful to understand the real norms and values of an organization's culture. Rituals are time-honored customs that enable individuals to understand social relationships by delineating the parameters that determine belonging or not belonging. "Rituals are used to create order, clarity, and predictability particularly in dealing with issues and problems that are too complex, mysterious, or random to be controlled in any other way . . . Individuals use rituals to reduce uncertainty and anxiety . . . Rituals serve four major functions: to socialize, to stabilize, to reduce ambiguity, and to convey messages to outsiders'' (Bolman and Deal 1984, pp. 158-159).

Some events or processes, considered legitimate and logical, are really only rituals. Consider the following outline by Bolman and Deal (1984, p. 162):

• Performance appraisals that may be simply pro-forma exercises but still are done religiously every year.

• Committee meetings that produce few results, waste a lot of time, but still are scheduled and attended.

• Training programs that produce few real performance results but are used to socialize participants or to provide a showcase for top brass.

Stories describe conflicts between organizational and personal needs. Stories also provide causal explanations for success and failure. Wilkins (1984) describes the relationship between stories and management philosophy. According to Wilkins, stories are powerful in passing on culture because they are like maps that help people know how things are done and why they are done. ``Stories become symbols for people. They are accounts of concrete events which can be examples of shared principles and purposes'' (Wilkins 1984, p. 45). Wilkins describes one company in which all of the employees knew the story of the company's refusal to lay off workers during a massive economic recession when all other industries were reducing their staff. This story is used as a symbol for the company's commitment to worker security and to reinforce the image of the company as ``having a heart'' (Wilkins 1984, pp. 46-47). Another company encourages circulation of stories about managers being ``beaten up'' when presenting new proposals or requests. These stories reinforce the norm of being tough and having to be able to "take it" if a manager wants to survive and succeed.

Like stories, myths, which entail a narrative of events in dramatic form, are also useful in establishing what is legitimate and what is acceptable. Myths anchor the present in the past, offer explanations, and therefore provide legitimacy for what is socially significant. Myths justify, sustain, explain and reconcile the contradictions and incongruities between professed values and actual behavior (Pettigrew 1979, p. 576). Myths can be helpful or destructive. They can keep us sane or they can blind us to reality. Myths explain, express, legitimize, and mediate contradictions. They help protect people from uncertainty but also can misdirect needed attention. Common myths in organizations include: authority must equal responsibility, happy workers are productive workers, hard work will be rewarded by promotion, and all problems have solutions. You just have to define the problem correctly.

It is not sufficient to have knowledge of the formal structure, the written rules and policies. These only represent the surface or the conscious life of the organization. Penetration beneath the surface level is necessary to understand the true reality of the organization, which consists of both the overt and the covert or the conscious and the unconscious. Linkage, among values, beliefs, and actions are often explained by the organization rituals, myths, and stories. A diverse sample of these and other indicators are necessary to form a true picture of an organization's culture.

Cultural Indicators

What are the indicators of an organization's culture? Elements of a culture include both informal rules, communication systems and styles, and rites and rituals. "Without expressive rites and events, any culture will die. In the absence of ceremony or ritual, important values have no impact" (Deal and Kennedy 1982, pp. 63-64). Some organizations have many rituals, some few, but they are always important. Rituals may include the company picnic, Christmas parties, the annual softball game, Friday afternoon beer busts or tea parties, the awards dinner, the 25-year club, bake sales, Thanksgiving turkeys, the yearly marathon, New Year's Day receptions, retirement parties or momentos, or Monday morning breakfast meetings. A ritual is any event that has significance to the organization and has been going on for a long time. Ignorance or noncompliance with rituals is generally noted and frowned upon by those in power.

Formal and informal rules that reflect the values and norms of the culture are those policies and customs related to dress, hair, intimacy, social decorum, status symbols, and the physical environment. Expectations for compliance with rules and customs are also a norm. In some organizational cultures strict compliance with custom is expected; in others one can be selective or inconsistent without penalty. For example, an organization may demand that male employees always wear jackets and ties but female employees can wear anything without censure. Or, employees that serve clients or patients directly must dress aseptically and aesthetically, while behind-the-scene employees can dress casually and informally. In the 1960s, hair length and style became a *cause celebre* in many organizations because of the popularity of the hippie or "Jesus" style on men. Even today there are formal or informal rules about facial hair and length of men's hair. Many books and articles have been written on the subject of dressing for success. The right look, however, whether in hair, makeup, clothing, or physical image, is the look that is both acceptable to those who count in the organization and congruent with organizational values.

Intimacy and social decorum norms refer to personal behavior as well as behavior between opposite sexes and between superiors and subordinates. Are physicians always addressed as "Doctor" while nurses and other women are addressed by first name? Are flirting, affectionate language and physical touching accepted or frowned upon? Who can dance with whom at the social events? Is any behavior tolerated as long as one is discreet? Is smoking or coffee drinking acceptable at the nurse's station or restricted to lounges? Is socializing off the job acceptable? If so, is it limited to peers, or can superiors and subordinates also socialize? Are there different behavioral expectations and norms for men and women?

There may be unwritten rules about work habits, such as how much time is allowed for goofing off, or how strictly lunch hours and starting and quitting times are observed. Some organizations have expectations or rules regarding status symbols, such as what kind of care subordinates and superiors should own or what kind of desk a manager can have. The location of parking spaces and offices are common status symbols and reflect norms and values related to power. White coats, stethoscopes, beepers, and personal desktop computers are also observable symbols of who has achieved status, who has power, and who is allowed to flaunt his or her success.

Rules and customs related to the physical environment include the presence of plants, flowers, artwork, personal belongings, or family pictures in the individual's work area. Must everyone comply with the company look, or is individuality the norm? Are there certain objects or colors that cannot be used? Is the physical setting spit-and-polish, elegant, seedy homey, modern, traditional, sterile, or a combination of the above? Are there spaces for employees to relax, eat, and socialize, or are all spaces used for organizational needs? Are there separate facilities for doctors and administration? Use and appearance of space are usually reliable indicators of the particular norms and values of an organization.

Another element identified as part of an organization's culture is the communication system or style. Communication systems include the formal channels of information flow as diagrammed on an organization chart, the annual reports, recruitment materials, personnel manuals, minutes of meetings, and publicity or advertising materials. These documents and materials illustrate the formality or informality of communication, the kind of information that is important, and the value placed on specificity or ambiguity of messages. In addition to the formal kinds of communication, there are always unwritten rules and customs for personal communication, which often occupies an amazing amount of people's time. There are norms related to the acceptance or nonacceptance of four-letter words, ethnic jokes, and jargon or double-talk. There are norms related to whether communications should be verbal or written and whether presentations should be slick or informal, long or short, written in prose style or terse outline. There may also be norms and customs related to who speaks first at a meeting, how much, if any, disagreement is tolerated, who laughs at whose jokes, and who has the last word.

Other norms and values of a culture relate to how strangers are treated and how long it takes before a newcomer becomes part of the "family." There may be unwritten or specific norms for the manager's involvement in community events and affairs as well as values related to the manager's family life, religious preferences, and political party affiliation. Although the norms and values of an organization may appear arbitrary, capricious, unfair, and even silly, without them it is hard to know how to behave. Such rules, rituals, and customs, as in any culture, let people know where they stand, reinforce one's place within an organization or society, and set the parameters for how people can relate to one another.

According to Deal and Kennedy (1982), an organization's culture also determines the roles individuals can play in addition to their occupational or job identification. Some of the roles they identify in their book *Corporate Cultures* include those of storyteller, priest, hero, whisperer, and gossip. Storytellers interpret what is going on, impart legends to new employees, know what it takes to get ahead, and have access to important information. Priests are guardians of the rituals and customs, listen to confession but don't tell, and fill you in on the historical perspective. Heroes are those who personify the organizational values and are the main characters in the legends. Whisperers are those who have the ear of the people in power and keep them informed of what is going on. Gossips pass on bad news or distort good news. They may not be close to power brokers but can serve a useful purpose. Organizations may also have one or more cabals, groups of individuals who secretly join forces and always support one another's position and arguments in public or in meetings.

Because of functional differences, gender differences, or socioeconomic and educational differences, all complex organizations also have subcultures. Some examples of subcultures within a hospital are physicians and nurses, accounting and housekeeping, the operating room and the mental health unit. Subcultures tend to come into conflict with one another, and these conflicts can lead to organizational dilemmas if the subculture's values or norms are incongruent with those of the overall culture. Conflict can be either healthy and promote innovation and problem solving or be destructive, halting productivity and compromising organizational success. How conflict is handled between and among subcultures will affect everyone's future success. Recognition of the differences between subcultures and encouragement of what each has to contribute can have positive effects and outcomes.

The organization itself is part of a larger context identified as the external environment or the community. The external environment influences the hospital in at least two major ways. First, the hospital is dependent upon the external environment for its patients, personnel, and supplies. Second, the hospital is affected by the characteristics and needs of the community. These characteristics include the age and sex composition of the individuals in the community, occupational skills and credentials of community residents, attitudes toward health and illness, expectations of health care providers, and the norms and values of minority and majority ethnic and cultural groups. All of those characteristics and variables comprise an interactive system which may be analyzed using a systems concept.

Systems concepts are directed toward providing a broad model for understanding all organizations. Contingency views, a subset of systems concepts, acknowledge that the environment and internal subsystems of each organization are somewhat unique and provide a basis for designing and managing specific organizations. An underlying assumption of the contingency view is that there should be congruence between the organization and its environment and among the various subsystems. Thus the primary managerial role is to maximize this congruence (Georgopoulos 1982, p. 31). Managing such congruence is particularly difficult when there is a need for innovation and change in an organization's culture in order to adapt to what is happening in the external environment. "Change always threatens culture. People form strong attachments to heroes, legends, the rituals of daily life, the hoopla of extravaganzas and ceremonies, all the symbols and settings of the work place. Change strips down these relationships and leaves employees confused, insecure and often angry . . . It can literally take years to achieve fundamental change in an organization's culture" (Deal and Kennedy 1982, p. 157).

Conclusion

Successful managers and executives are not born or just lucky. They are sensitive, knowledgeable, and hard-working. Successful managers and executives are sensitive to the organization's norms and values and to individual's needs, vested interests, and hidden agendas. Successful managers and executives learn the available technical, interpersonal, and political skills and know when they will be relevant and congruent in the organization. Successful managers and executives work hard at using their technical, interpersonal, and political skills, learning from both their successes and their failures. Successful managers and executives have a sense of timing for events and nuances, acting when the timing is right and holding back when the timing is wrong.

Last but not least, successful managers and executives have a healthy sense of humor and a well-developed sense of the ridiculous. Successful managers can laugh at both themselves and the situation. As has been said,

> Among the animals, one has a sense of humor. Humor saves a few steps, it saves years.
>
> Marianne Moore, "The Pangolin"

An Organizational Culture Checklist

What beliefs and norms organize and influence rules, policies, and behavior in your organization? What is the desired image? What is explicit and what is implicit? The following checklist is neither all-inclusive nor universally applicable. It may be helpful, however, for learning about and understanding your organization's culture and subcultures.

Image

- How does the organization wish to be perceived? What word, slogans, or phrases are used in describing the organization? Examples: friendly, caring, innovative, safe, up and coming, biggest, oldest, dependable.
- Is money obviously being spent on creating this image with respect to decor, landscaping, equipment, signage, public relation activities, annual reports, or community activities?
- How does the public get access to the organization? Through a lobby, parking garage, clinic, or reception area? How comfortable, attractive, and secure is this access?
- How are visitors treated? Does the treatment depend on socioeconomic status?
- Is community involvement expected of employees? If so, does it depend on position or status in the organization?

Deportment

• Is there a dress code? How strictly is it enforced? Is it different for men and women? Do people dress formally/informally? Does this depend on status in the hierarchy?

• Is facial hair tolerated on men? Is hair length or style an issue? How much makeup and jewelry can women wear?

• Is touching acceptable or desirable? Only between same-sex employees or between opposite sexes? How much, if any, affection is acceptable?

• What kind of relationships are acceptable off the job between different sexes, at different job or position levels?

• Can people "let themselves go" at parties or social events?

• Is social drinking or smoking acceptable on the job?

• Are there off-limits places for employees?

• Does it matter whom you hang around with or does it depend on your position?

• Are there social stratifications? If so, what is the basis of this stratification: title, department, personal relationship?

• Is swearing or use of four-letter words acceptable? Can employees tell off-color or ethnic jokes?

• Do employees use first names or last names with each other? Does it depend on job position or gender? Does it depend on the setting, e.g., social gatherings versus work?

• Are sexist behaviors tolerated? Does it depend on title or status?

Status Symbols and Reward Systems

• Are there any acknowledged symbols of status such as space, titles, or special privileges?

• On what basis are promotions given: performance, longevity, loyalty? Are upper-level positions given to outsiders or only to those who have "earned their stripes"?

- Are there restricted areas or areas that are off-limits except for special groups, such as meeting rooms or lounge spaces?

- Do only specific individuals or positions warrant reserved parking or personal bathrooms or closets?

- What are the elitist committees, societies, projects, or events?

- Do certain people receive special perquisites such as a company car, country club membership, or professional association dues? Who are those individuals?

- What badges or physical indicators such as beepers, personal desktop computers, different uniforms, or clipboards set people apart as being special?

- Who gets sent to the fun cities for conventions and meetings?

- Do titles truly reflect status and authority in the organization?

Environment and Ambiance

- Are there lounges or places for employees to relax? Where are they located? How attractive and comfortable are they?

- Are eating and drinking allowed in the work area?

- Are there public eating areas? Who has access? What is the appearance and ambiance?

- Can employees have plants, photographs, posters, or other individual touches in their work area or offices?

- Is there a company color scheme? If so, is it subdued, bright, sterile?

- Is music provided or acceptable in work areas or offices?

- What are the norms in regard to starting time, quitting time, and "goof-off" time?

- Who eats with whom? Are there separate eating areas for special groups?

• How is office furniture arranged? Is open seating at tables or in a circle encouraged?

Communication

• Is the norm for important communication verbal or written?

• Are written communications formal or informal? Is the preferred style narrative or memo? Is language to the point or circuitous?

• Is jargon acceptable or desirable? In the organization? with clients or outsiders?

• Are minutes of meetings kept? Are they circulated? If so, to whom? What kind of reports are important and what kind are filed in the wastebasket?

• Is rumor the usual method of information distribution?

• Are there bulletin boards, company newsletters, or house organs? How important or meaningful are these means of communication? What is their purpose: recognition, information, or both?

• Does important information flow from the top down or from the bottom up? Can the chain of command be circumvented without punishment?

• Where does important communication take place: in meetings, in the hall, at social functions, away from the place of business, in the men's room?

Meetings

• Are there unwritten rules about who speaks first and last at meetings?

• What meetings can you skip without being punished or missing anything important?

- Is it permissible to come late or leave early, or does it depend on whose meeting it is?

- Where are people seated? Are there territorial rights? Are there established arrangements based on status or hierarchy?

- Is discussion allowed? Is the agenda predetermined and no adjustments permissible?

- Are refreshments provided? Who pours or serves the refreshments? Does everyone help himself?

- Are time limits strictly enforced?

Rites, Rituals, and Ceremonies

- Are there established rituals that must be attended, such as Monday morning executive breakfast meetings, Friday afternoon drinks or beer bashes, Christmas parties, the annual picnic?

- Is orientation to the organization special? Who greets new employees? Is orientation different for different position levels?

- What does the organization do to recognize length of service? birth of employees' children? retirement? marriage? death in employees' families?

- Are there sports teams? How important is membership or participation?

- Are there rules or assumptions about how long you have to be employed before you are considered an insider?

Sacred Cows

(A sacred cow is a person, place, thing, or belief that cannot be discussed, attacked, or ignored. Sacred cows are revered and protected. Denial of the existence of sacred cows or failure to give fealty to them is fraught with risk.)

- Are there heroes, living or dead, in the organization who are revered and honored? How did these individuals get to be heroes?

- Are there any myths about he organization that must be perpetuated, such as, "We have a mission to the poor and needy"?

- Are there any subjects or ideas that are taboo, such as unionization or merit systems?

- Are there rules or policies that are sacrosanct and cannot be changed even if outdated, ineffective, or illogical?

- Are there relationships between departments, individuals, or groups that cannot be threatened, challenged, or questioned, such as between physicians and nurses or between lay members and professional or religious members of the board?

- If there is a difference between what we do and what we say, is it acceptable to acknowledge this inconsistency or is it taboo to suggest that such a situation even exists?

- Can employees speak freely to the media or are all public relations and statements carefully controlled?

Subcultures

- Are there any? If so, what purpose do they serve? Is the purpose deliberate?

- If there are subcultures are they subrosa or overt? Are they tolerated or pointed to with pride as our unique group, department, or unit?

PART II

Case Studies

case study 1

Playing the game

SETTING AND EXTERNAL ENVIRONMENT

The setting for this case is a large acute care hospital with over 4000 employees in a large city in the western United States. The hospital, a not-for-profit voluntary agency, is well established in the community and has served a changing population for many years. Once a predominantly middle-class neighborhood, the community is now a mix of lower socioeconomic residents, immigrants from Asia, and a core of professional middle-class families. This neighborhood mix is reflected in the reimbursement sources, which is one-third indigent, one-third private insurers, and one-third Medicare.

There is little industry in the area except for service businesses such as restaurants, small shops, and family-owned enterprises. A nearby large university with a medical school uses the hospital facilities for education and research. Various nursing schools also use the hospital for clinical practice both on the inpatient service and in the very busy clinic services.

Control of the hospital is vested in a Board of Directors representing the middle-class community, the university, hospital management, and some outsiders with good connections or famous names. The Board has recently voted to establish a holding company, which will be organized as for-profit, in order to promote some new services and to take over some neighborhood facilities such as a physician's clinic and a geriatric center. A more entrepreneurial approach to doing business is perceived as the way to go in a newly competitive environment.

Particularly worrisome is the large indigent population, which the hospital feels a moral obligation to serve but which is a financial drain. Any venture that will increase the private-paying percentage of patients or bring in additional revenue is encouraged and subsidized.

Internal Environment

The metaphors used by insiders to describe the organization are mixed. Some people call it a "jungle," while others describe it as a "special" place. Top management would like the organization to be perceived as up-and-coming and trendsetting. The predominant management style is aggressive and confrontational. Managers are expected to be producers and to get results, but at the same time be responsive to individual needs. *In Search of Excellence* is required reading for all middle and top management. These two groups are predominantly white Anglo-Saxon while first-line management is a mix of orientals, chicanos, blacks, and caucasians. Everyone is on a first-name basis with the exception of the new Corporate President, who is addressed as "Mr." First-line and middle managers are selected on the basis of competence and loyalty. Higher management positions go to those who know how to play internal and external political games within the organization. Who is aligned with whom is crucial to success. A new manager must be astute in the choice of friends and allies. Academic credentials and credibility or renown in the outside world are perceived as very desirable and are rewarded within the organization.

The organizational structure is centralized and many-tiered. This structure is somewhat of a contradiction to the new entrepreneurial spirit, but relinquishing the power inherent to a line structure is unthinkable at this point. Long-range goals and strategic planning are highly touted, but except for the achievement of immediate objectives, means to an end are more important and more obviously the focus of activity. Communication patterns are very informal. An efficient, effective, reliable grapevine operates throughout the entire organization. Little is written or recorded. Everyone depends on and uses verbal methods to pass on information, and this system works extremely well considering the size of the organization.

Most employees are well-credentialed. Formal education is highly valued and supported with tuition assistance, educational leaves, and paid attendance at educational conferences. Upward mobility is encouraged and is a part of all union contracts. Formalized in-service training or staff development is provided for nursing department employees only. Other departments use an on-the-job training approach. Promotion is both from within and from the outside. "The best person for the job" is an ethic both preached and practiced. Although employee satisfaction and high morale are posited as organizational goals, employees are treated inconsistently--as adults one day and children the next. Part of this inconsistency may be attributed to the presence of several labor unions, which demand and get strict adherence to contractual terms.

Although the predominant management style is aggressive and confrontational, administration is adamant that managers either have an open-door policy or be always available to employees. This sometimes causes considerable frustration for managers, who can get sidetracked or delayed from tasks by the need to respond instantly to an employee's problems. Several managers including the Director of Nursing have had to establish an appointment or available-hours policy in order to avoid the constant interruptions.

Rule compliance is not an important issue, nor is control except when it relates to political or financial matters. Managers are expected to adhere to union contracts in order to avoid grievances, but when it is possible, they are rewarded for being flexible. Dress code is practically nonexistent, and everyone is casual in appearance. Occasionally patients complain they can't tell who anyone is, but this is dealt with on an individual basis. Personnel pride themselves on getting positive satisfaction ratings from patients and try to live up to the hospital's image of being warm and "homey." To some extent,

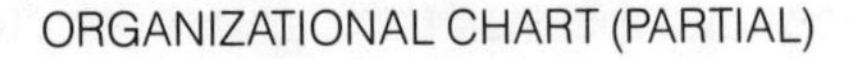
ORGANIZATIONAL CHART (PARTIAL)

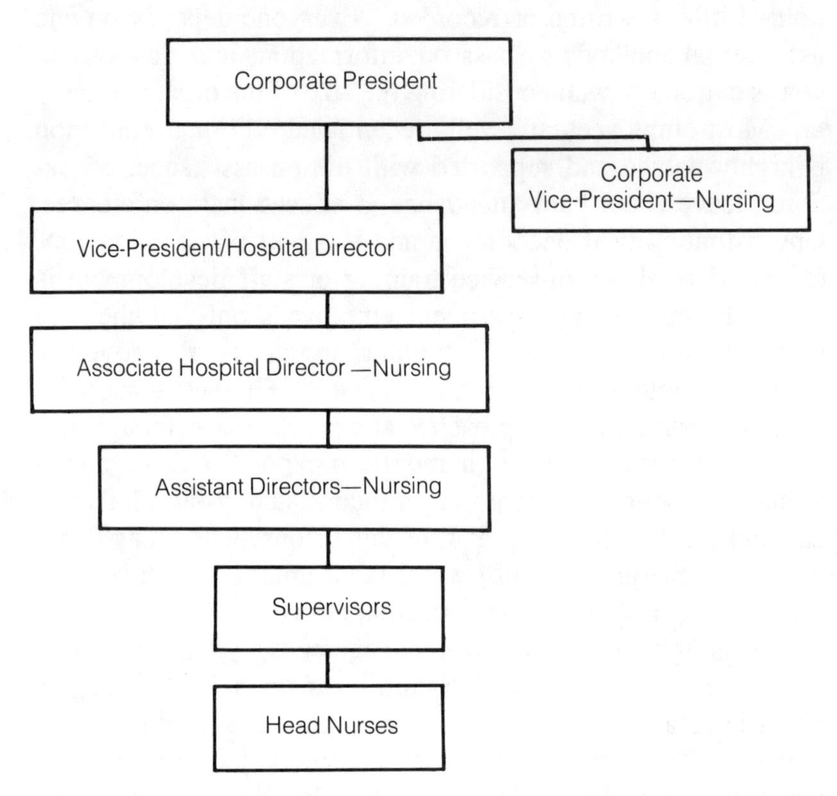

nursing staff carries this emphasis on "being nice" to an extreme, with subsequent criticism by some about the quality or standard of care.

There are few rituals or heroes in the organization. A few old-timers know the history and try to preserve the myths, but administration has little interest in the past since they were not part of it. Instead there is expressed impatience and a "let's get on with it" attitude. In fact, many of the newer management people would like to wipe out the past history of the organization. Status is based on political alignments and friendships, not on office size, location, or furnishings. Rank does have its privileges but not in an overwhelmingly obvious way. Titles are meaningful, particularly since there are so many layers in the organizational chart.

Nursing, prior to the arrival of the Director of Nursing, was perceived as somewhat of a subculture or stepchild. The department was tolerated out of necessity but was not considered terribly credible or as having much influence. This lack of status was partially related to previous directors' lack of powerful connections. The department is well staffed by most standards and over the years has been able to convert to an almost all-RN complement in the most acute areas. Recruitment is an ongoing need because of the urban location, but generally positions are filled without too long a delay. Because of continual turnover, orientation and staff development consume a great deal of time, and any efforts that increase retention time are highly rewarded.

Approximately half of the nursing management group have been there for many years, having risen from the ranks. The other half are a mixture of people hired by one or the other past directors of nursing. Most managers are competent but have not been assertive in advancing nursing's status within the organization. Except for a few individuals, they could be described as well-meaning but politically naive.

Principal Players and Supporting Characters

Vice-President Hospital Director (VPHD)

The VPHD, in his middle 50s, is an up-from-the-ranks oldtimer. He has lots of ties to the powerful and semi-powerful. A 20-year veteran of the system, he knows how to play the games and plays them well. He gets things done because he is aligned with the right people, but he does not flaunt his connections. He is generally liked by his subordinates and has a good reputation as a community person. He is supportive of the Associate Hospital Director--Nursing and his other associate directors but never loses sight of the political realities of power.

Associate Hospital Director--Nursing (AHDN)

This position, one of five associate directors positions at the hospital, has been filled by a succession of three women over the past ten years. The individual in place at the time of the incident described here is, like her predecessors, an outsider entering her first top job in nursing administration. Unlike the others, she is somewhat older, in her early 40s. The current AHDN was hired by the previous VPHD personally after only one interview. No search committee or nursing input on the selection was solicited. The AHDN is well-credentialed, with excellent references and an active background in regional nursing associations. Her practice background was in prestigious organizations. Her previous administrative experience consisted of less than two years as a middle manager. However, she and the previous VPHD, a credible, competent, political outsider whose tenure at the hospital was brief, had an immediate positive relationship, and he believed she could do the job. Described by colleagues as "warm and wonderful," the AHDN believed herself to be politically savvy but realized somewhat late that she was still a bit of a "babe in the woods."

The AHDN has worked vigorously and successfully at establishing ties and recognition in the community.

Corporate Vice-President--Nursing (CVPN)

The CVPN, hired directly by the Corporate President, is a strong, extremely well-credentialed, attractive woman in her 40s. She is described as very bright, very savvy, and very accomplished. She has a national reputation and is part of an extensive professional network of the famous and would-be-famous.

The CVPN's role was never clearly defined within or outside the organization. A job description was never written, nor were her duties and responsibilities clearly outlined. On the organizational chart, the CVPN reports directly to the Corporate President and has no line authority. She preferred to see the position evolve as she became more familiar with the community and the organization.

Background

Although the AHDN was hired before the arrival of the CVPN, she was well-informed about the latter position and the possibility of the incumbent taking the job. The AHDN understood the organizational relationship to be that shown on the organizational chart. Her understanding was that CVPN would be a consultant to her, with no line authority. The AHDN believed that the CVPN's national reputation and experience in financial management as well as strategic planning would be of great help to her, as these were skills the AHDN had not yet developed. The AHDN also was very much involved in changing the nursing department's status within the organization and thus was somewhat relieved to know there would be someone she could call upon for assistance in the other areas.

The AHDN moved slowly but vigorously within her own department. She began to build her own team by shifting individuals she felt were not team players to other positions. She purposely did not terminate anyone but tried to help them find a mutually desirable place in the organization. She hoped these strategies would result in a team of effective and loyal members. At the same time she made clear that she expected her group to "clean up their act" and hold staff accountable for a high standard of patient care. The AHDN believed she had made considerable progress toward her two goals of improving nursing's status in the organization and upgrading the quality of care. Several other non-nurse administrators agreed with her and were very supportive of her efforts.

Initially, all went well between the CVPN and the AHDN. They met on a regular basis and seemed to agree on goals for the nursing department and on most of the means to these ends. The AHDN helped the CVPN meet both lay and professional people in the community. The CVPN also was very busy helping the administration weed out people who were considered undesirable from the organizational perspective. She also quickly grasped who were the power players and made sure she became aligned with them. It was conceded by others that the CVPN was a master at win-lose strategies.

Several months after the CVPN's arrival, the AHDN began to feel something was amiss. She became aware of grapevine gossip to the effect that she was trying to undermine the CVPN's position. In her perception this was not true, and therefore, she met with the CVPN to clear the air. This confrontation seemed to achieve that objective and all went well for another few months.

The Incident

After a several-month hiatus, the AHDN is once more at odds with the CVPN. She is called on the carpet over a medication error study she initiated in an attempt to both establish a practice standard and involve the staff in nursing research. The CVPN has implied to the Corporate President that the rate is far too high, is dangerous, and is indicative of the AHDN's poor nursing administration. The CVPN also implies that she is purposely being kept in the dark by the AHDN.

At the same time these events are occurring, the AHDN realizes that information shared only in her administrative meetings is being leaked to the CVPN. The AHDN suspects a spy, but cannot identify the culprit. In an attempt to resolve the two "misunderstandings," the AHDN goes to her boss, the VPHD, who advises her to keep a low profile. He is willing to support her but not at the price of antagonizing powerful players. While still attempting to resolve the issue of the medication error study with win-win strategies, the AHDN is faced with two new crises. The CVPN is furious because the AHDN will not support a clinical ladder concept, one favored and recommended by the CVPN to increase retention. She accuses the AHDN of undermining her once more by discussing her objections at a management meeting. The CVPN also forbids the AHDN to extend the "two-day alternative" plan, a concession the AHDN has promised the union delegates based on their request and a survey of collective bargaining unit members.

Once more, the AHDN goes to the VPHD, who observes that she and the CVPN don't seem to be able to work together. Although he does not force the issue, the AHDN believes she is getting a strong message and submits her resignation, effective that same day.

Questions

1. Could the situation leading to the resignation have been avoided or somehow changed?

2. Was AHDN a "babe in the woods," or were there other unresolvable or unpreventable factors operating in the organization?

case study 2

A case of double messages

Setting and External Environment

The case takes place in a 500-bed acute care hospital located in a suburban southeastern community. The present facility is only four years old. There are also older buildings that have been renovated from the original 50-year-old construction. The hospital, a nonprofit, freestanding facility, is contemplating the addition of a new pediatric division even though there are two well-known children's hospitals within 25 miles.

The hospital has served the community's routine medical care needs for over 50 years. Patients with complex problems have always been sent to the big city. The new administration wants to change this practice and establish the hospital as a tertiary care center. This hospital with three other small community hospitals is aggressively pursuing a consortium of services that can be marketed in competition with the urban medical center. There is extreme optimism about this venture, and there are high hopes for a revitalization of the surrounding area as a center for new industries and services.

The hospital was previously managed by a board selected from the community; a reformed Board of Trustees now includes out-of-towners who perceive that management should have more day-to-day control. Historically, the hospital has been fiscally sound. However, economic changes in the surrounding community have affected the hospital patient population, which is now heavily Medicare/Medicaid. Although utilization continues high, bad debt has increased and fiscal matters occupy much of management's time and discussions.

The external environment has changed considerably over the last 20 years. The two or three major industries that employed a large number of people have moved out, resulting in a rather high unemployment rate. At the same time expansion of the nearby urban center has brought a large number of professionals who work in the city but wish to enjoy the benefits of suburbia. These people are described as nouveau riche by old-time residents, who are predominantly white Anglo-Saxon or Protestant. A large number of poor Spanish-speaking people have also immigrated to the area, attracted by the climate and the availability of sporadic work.

Internal Environment

Historically, the environment of the organization was best described as one big, happy family. Many employees were related to one another. Superficially, everyone was informal and used first names, even with physicians. However, employees were also expected to know their place and observe certain norms of behavior, such as in dress--uniforms were expected of all nurses--and respect for authority.

In the past, credentials were not important. Managers came up from the ranks after serving their time, and then became members of an exclusive boys' club--the Director of Nursing was not included. Promotion was exclusively from within. This situation has changed with the advent of the new Board of Trustees configuration. The Chief Operating Officer and the Chief Executive Officer are the first non-Protestant, noninsiders to hold these positions. Both are highly credentialed. The Chief Executive Officer is also the first nonphysician to head the management team. Suddenly there is a new image among managers, with three-piece suits and attache cases much in evidence. Even nurse managers now wear street clothes. Many managers are busy signing up for degree and nondegree courses to meet new expectations for their positions.

There are a number of double messages being given by the new management. One is innovation, but not too vigorous. Another is accountability, but don't create conditions that may favor union activity. Although long-term planning is touted, short-term outcomes are rewarded. Many new rules and policies have been developed, but most deal with trivial concerns. Important issues are submerged in a high level of busyness.

Communication continues to be informal, with tacit approval of bypassing the formal system to find out what you need or to inform those who need to be informed. Most real business takes place in hallways or at meals. Memos are infrequent and minutes of meetings rarely kept or distributed. The past warm and positive ambiance has been replaced by a feeling that too much is happening too fast. There has been an increase in rumors among staff, and many employees who are still of the old culture express uneasiness and a need to "tell them what they want to hear but do what you've always done."

Principal Players and Supporting Characters

Chief Executive Officer (CEO)

The CEO, an outsider and newcomer, is in his middle 30s. He has been married twice and has several young children. Master's-prepared he is both socially and professionally ambitious. This is his first position as CEO and he wants it to be a success so he can move later to a more prestigious position. Bright and charming, the CEO has as one of his main objectives to establish himself with the movers and shakers in the community. He hired both the Chief Operating Officer and the Director of Marketing, a new position that reports directly to him. The CEO knows the Vice-President for Nursing from another institution where they both worked. He is supportive in a distant, formal way and insists that the Vice-President for

Nursing observe the established chain of command. The CEO maintains minimal social relationships with his management team but intense outside activity with certain members of the Board. He continuously stresses the importance of bottom-line results but is also very conscious of power relationships.

Chief Operating Officer (COO)

The COO, also a new, master's-prepared outsider, is in his early 40s. He is described as an effective middle manager who has been promoted beyond his level of competence. He is not ambitious and is very traditional in his perception of nurses' role. For example, he doesn't know why nurses need a baccalaureate degree or why LPNs can't be used in the operating room as both scrub and circulating nurses. The Vice-President for Nursing was his personal choice as director of nursing. Until the incident related, he was supportive of her activities and objectives.

Vice-President for Nursing (VPN)

The VPN is a divorced woman in her middle 40s. She is the only newcomer who is also a white, Anglo-Saxon Protestant. This is her first job as a Vice-President of Nursing, although she had many years of experience as an associate director and as a supervisor. Although this new position required a change of environment where she knew everyone and all the organizational norms for a foreign territory and new organization culture, she felt the time was right. She has put most of her energy into the job and has had little opportunity to establish herself in the community except with other nursing directors. She is a nonvoting member of several medical committees.

Supervisor: Critical Care Units (SCCU)

SCCU is a married woman in her late 30s who is an old-guard member of both the hospital and the community. Most of her professional life has been spent in this hospital. She is currently working on a baccalaureate degree, but not in nursing. Prior to being promoted to this position, a new one created by the VPN, she was a head nurse in one of the intensive care units. She has been made chairperson of the practice committee by the VPN and interacts well with the intensive care physicians. The SCCU is pleasant and capable but is especially concerned about being liked by her staff.

Vice President for Human Resources (VPHR)

The VPHR, in his late 30s, was brought in from the outside four years ago by the then-executive officer. Described as a "Mister Nice Guy," he gives lots of lip service to policies and rules but in reality does what is most expedient and least risky. Although he is on the executive team he has little real relationship with the good old boys. He is sensitive, however, to political nuances and where power lies.

Background

Many changes have occurred in the management of the hospital over the past 18 months. A new, centralized reporting system has been established and leaves the CEO free from everyday operating decisions. Fiscal responsibility has become the party line, and everyone has been informed about the importance of budgeting and cost containment.

At the same time, many other things stay the same. Although both staff and first-line managers are expected to be financially accountable, no efforts have been made to train or educate them for these responsibilities. There is little staff development, even in the nursing department, and no one except vice-presidents goes to outside meetings or continuing education events.

The new VPN, hired 12 months ago to replace the retiring director, has made the development of head nurses one of her

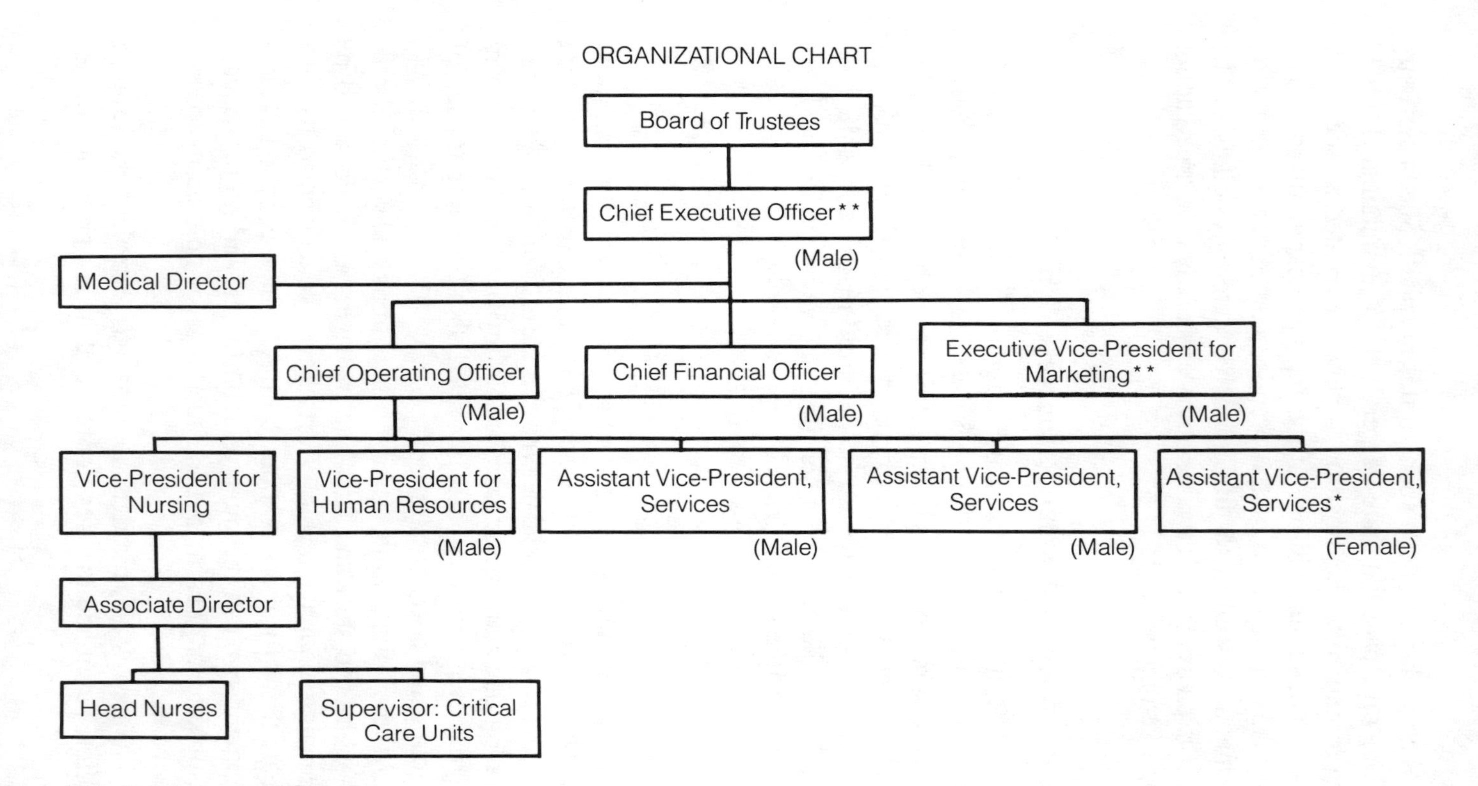
ORGANIZATIONAL CHART
Board of Trustees
Chief Executive Officer**
(Male)
Medical Director
Chief Operating Officer
(Male)
Chief Financial Officer
(Male)
Executive Vice-President for Marketing**
(Male)
Vice-President for Nursing
Vice-President for Human Resources
(Male)
Assistant Vice-President, Services
(Male)
Assistant Vice-President, Services
(Male)
Assistant Vice-President, Services*
(Female)
Associate Director
Head Nurses
Supervisor: Critical Care Units
** = Newcomer and Outsider
* = Newcomer but Insider

goals. To this end she has flattened the organization chart, with head nurses reporting directly to the Associate Director. She created the SCCU position, replacing three head nurse positions. Previous supervisors were transferred to other positions or voluntarily retired. A structure of committees and task forces has been to work on standards of care and discuss contentious issues such as staffing.

Nursing administration is located in the same area as other administrators but occupies a very tiny space originally planned for social service. There are no conference rooms anywhere for nurses, nor are there any classrooms for educational functions.

After six months in the position, the VPN was appalled to find out that the person she believed was competently dealing with budget control was out of his depth and that nursing's budget was out of control. Although staffing was generally adequate, there was uncontrolled use of supplementary staff because of poor planning and no forecasting. Although all areas were out of line, the intensive care units were the worst. They were over budget for both staff and supplies. Investigation of this situation showed that the critical care nurses had established their own staffing norms. Since nights were perceived as undesirable, supplementary staff were used almost exclusively to cover this shift at a cost of $500,000. The Baylor Plan was used to cover weekends, with nurses receiving 40 hours pay for 24 hours of work as well as overtime to give report. All of the nurses who worked this plan had been doing so by choice for several years. Initiated because of a staffing shortage, the practice continued even though other nurses were willing to work a regular every-other-weekend off rotation.

The VPN called a conference with all the head nurses, the Associate Director, and the SCCU. She presented the facts and the responsibility for bringing the budget into line. Each manager was held responsible for submitting a plan for achieving this goal. All units submitted reasonable plans except for the critical care area, whose supervisor felt she couldn't change the staffing patterns.

The Incident

The VPN, believing that all units should meet the standards for meeting budget limitations, told the SCCU that she would have to reduce the use of supplementary nurses or replace it with an in-house pool and change the practice of covering weekends by the Baylor Plan. The SCCU was very reluctant to do this because of the staff's preference and satisfaction with the current arrangements.

At the same time that this was going on, the VPN was told to come to the COO's office, where he criticized her soundly for actions she had taken establishing a self-governance committee. Her perceived this as an action undermining the administration's authority and even encouraging collective bargaining activity. The VPN assured him that his committee was really working on standards of practice, something that was lacking in the nursing department.

Three days later the VPN had to take a week's personal leave because of a death in the family. While she was away someone leaked a story to the local paper about the proposed staffing changes in the critical care units and implied that these changes would severely limit nursing care and endanger patients' lives. The VPHR called a conference with the nurses from the critical care units about staffing and working conditions. Many complaints about the VPN, most of them groundless, were aired. The SCCU was not present at this meeting but was informed about it before it was held.

On her return to the hospital, the VPN was again summoned to the COO's office and asked to submit her resignation because "she no longer fit in with the administrative philosophy." Two days latter the SCCU was asked to be the Acting Vice-President for Nursing. She declined on the basis of a lack of appropriate credentials for the position.

Questions

1. Where did the VPN go wrong?

2. Are there any strategies she could have used to prevent the incident, or was it inevitable?

case study 3

Friends in high places

SETTING

This case takes place in a 250-bed nonprofit acute care hospital in an urban setting. Housed in an old, six-story high-rise building, the hospital has a very old history. Originally located further south in the city, its original mission was to provide public health services for immigrant women and children. The hospital now serves the acute care needs of both men and women of all age groups. Although the facilities are old, with the exception of a new, 15-bed intensive care unit, it is well maintained and attractive. All patient rooms are either private or semiprivate accommodations painted in soft pastels with new furniture. The pediatric unit is especially cheerful and homey-looking.

Funding for hospital services is divided about equally between federal/state reimbursement and private insurers. There is an intern-resident program associated with a medical school, although most of the incumbents are foreign and speak English as a second language. This situation causes some communication problems with both patients and nursing staff. The hospital has a reputation in the community for providing satisfactory care--not good, not bad. Recently, in response to numerous patient complaints of staff rudeness, several thousand dollars was spent on an attitude training program.

External Environment

The community in which the hospital is located has changed considerably over its many years. Originally a community of middle Europeans, it is now predominantly Asiatic and West Indian. There is a small middle-class white enclave and an alarmingly large number of drug users and dealers. The neighborhood is considered dangerous after dark, and drug-related crimes are frequent.

The hospital's primary competitor, a 700-bed medical center, is located directly across the street. This medical center has been quite successful in attracting a large private-paying clientele and is eroding the business of the smaller hospital. What keeps the hospital going is the presence of a very active Board of Trustees, composed primarily of very wealthy women. These women, direct descendants of the hospital's original Board, are very loyal to the hospital and take a day-to-day interest in what goes on, making frequent on-site rounds. The Chairperson of the Board, who is extremely wealthy, talks about "her hospital" and has frequently subsidized financial deficits out of her own fortune.

Internal Environment

The management of the hospital reflects the values and norms of the original community and the Board of Trustees. All managers are of Irish or Italian background, predominantly males who are very careful to take care of the Board's vested interests. The communication style is formal with everyone addressed by proper title and last name. Rewards and promotions come from belonging to the right ethnic and cultural group and maintaining the status quo. Management style is one of dealing with crisis rather than preventive problem solving or long-range planning. There is a great deal of frustration among the few managers hired from the outside who are considered competent and who want to "straighten the place out."

Interdepartmental problems are kicked upstairs, where they are ignored or dealt with superficially.

The majority of staff are Asiatic or black and reflect the values and norms of the more recent community population. Rumors and gossip are the usual method of communication, and a great deal of time is spent on discussing the latest "incident." Rules and policies are arbitrarily enforced and applied. There are no rituals followed by everyone except for an ethnic Christmas party, which was initiated by staff and is a big event for them. Management does not participate except for eating the various kinds of ethnic foods brought in by staff.

There is no management training and there are no staff education/development programs. No money is spent for outside continuing education or attendance at conventions and meetings. The ancillary personnel, many of them old-timers and unionized, feel they are treated paternalistically by most managers.

The nursing department, as part of a centralized organization, is somewhat top-heavy (see organizational chart). The Director of Nursing, on paper, reports to the Hospital Administrator, but in reality rarely sees him and is not part of his regular executive meetings. The Director of Nursing has no determination in her budget and knows only what she is told by the fiscal officer. Consequently, there is a lot of financial game-playing particularly with nursing positions, which turn over frequently. The Director of Nursing often hires nurses and then delays or postpones their arrival because of lack of funds. As a result, staffing is chronically short on the units. This situation coupled with inconsistent availability of supplies leads to considerable frustration in the nursing ranks.

The nursing staff is composed primarily of aides and RNs, with a few LPNs. Many of the nurses are foreign-born and are hired simply because they are available or because they are friends or relatives of other nurses or resident physicians. Functional nursing is the usual method of delivering care, although the staff education department is trying to introduce the team concept.

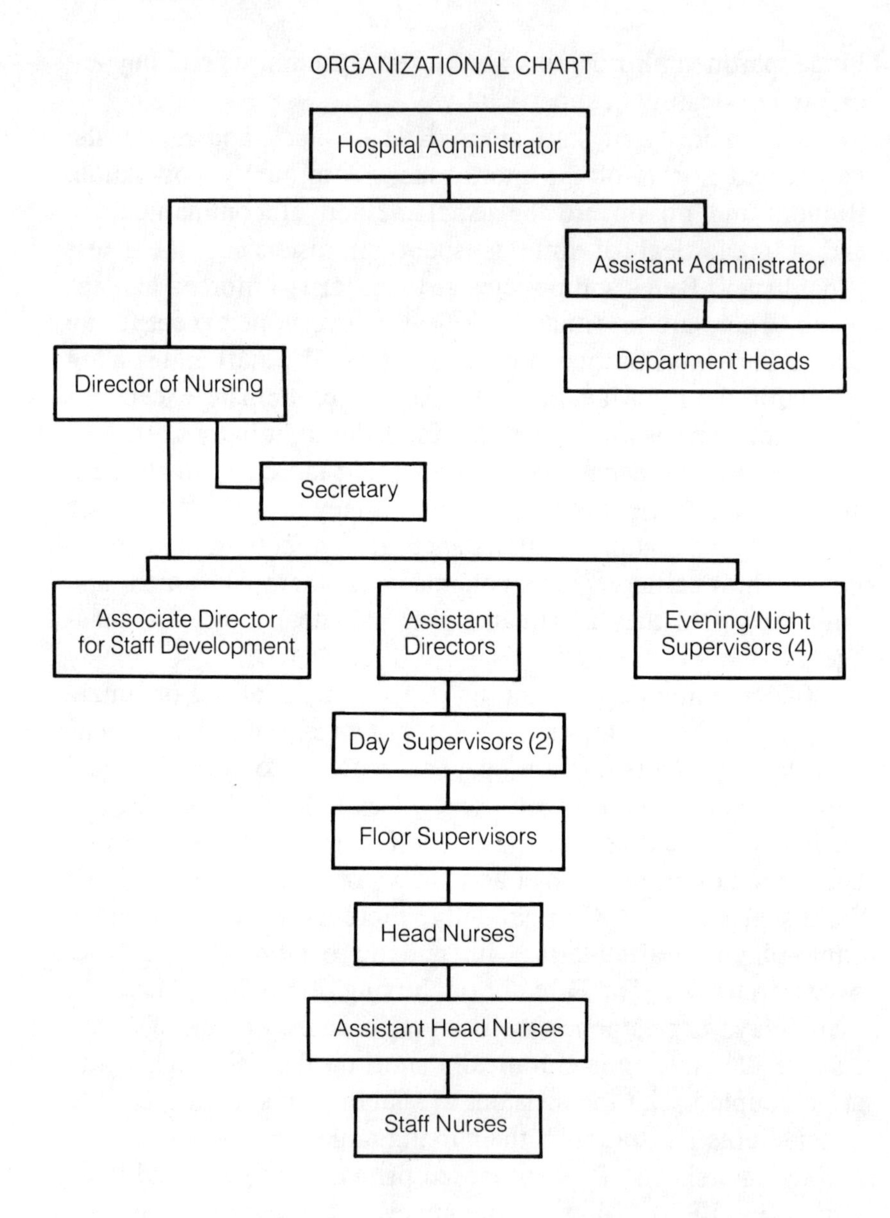
ORGANIZATIONAL CHART
Hospital Administrator
Assistant Administrator
Department Heads
Director of Nursing
Secretary
Associate Director for Staff Development
Assistant Directors
Evening/Night Supervisors (4)
Day Supervisors (2)
Floor Supervisors
Head Nurses
Assistant Head Nurses
Staff Nurses

Supervisors are, with one exception, old-timers and white. There is one supervisor for every floor, which is composed of one 45-bed unit managed by a head nurse and an assistant head nurse. Because of chronic staff shortages, the head nurse and the assistant usually end up doing patient care, so the supervisor in essence runs the floor. There are few standards of care, and little evaluation of performance is given. What the doctor says is usually the guiding principle for what is done to and for the patient.

PRINCIPAL PLAYERS AND SUPPORTING CHARACTERS

Hospital Administrator (HA)

Described as a figurehead, the HA is a man in his late 50s who has served as administrator for 20 years. Most of the work is done by his Assistant Administrator, whom he hired two years ago from the outside. The HA does pretty much what he is told to do by the Board. His style is one of avoidance whenever possible. He has irregular management meetings and for the most part lets his assistant, a younger, more committed person, handle the situation.

Director of Nursing (DON)

A single woman in her early 50s, the DON was hired 15 years ago from the outside. She does have a master's degree in nursing administration earned 25 years ago, but she does not keep up with trends or current concepts in nursing. She and one of the day supervisors are good friends, and both live in hospital housing down the block. The DON is described as incompetent, jovial, and friendly, addressing everyone by name. Her typical day consists of reading the two local daily newspapers, discussing last night's activities with her Assistant Director, and interviewing potential staff nurses. She is very close with her secretary, who does the DON's grocery shopping on company time and also irons and mends the DON's clothes in her office.

The DON has a poor relationship with the HA, who calls her only to convey complaints or problems. When the DON needs something she goes to the Assistant Administrator or the head of finance.

The DON has an excellent, long-standing personal relationship with one of the Board members closest to the Chairperson. Although the DON and this Board member do not mix socially, the DON visits her regularly on request in her apartment, bringing her food and medicine from the hospital kitchen and pharmacy.

Chairperson of the Board (COB)

The COB is an extremely wealthy widow in her 60s. She comes from an old family that has been associated with the hospital since its founding. The COB's money and family connections give her access to all the political powers in the city, which she uses for the hospital's benefit. The COB is a kind person who truly cares about the hospital, but she expects people to respond when she makes a request and feels that management really works for her. As indicated, she often subsidizes hospital deficits from her own fortune.

Associate Director for Staff Development (ADSD)

A single woman in her early 30s, the ADSD was hired by the DON about a year prior to the incident. She has previous experience as a supervisor, but this is her first position as a director of education, a newly created position in the nursing department. The ADSD is somewhat naive, believing that competence and high performance are the keys to organizational success. She is distressed about the quality of nursing care and is determined to help improve it. Her first six months on the job were spent developing the procedure manual, an audit plan, and a documentation system to meet Joint Commission on

Accreditation of Hospitals requirements. She is now working on an orientation and development program for newly hired nurses and has gotten permission to hire two instructors. The ADSD has become disenchanted with the DON's lack of leadership but gets along with her. The DON has neither interfered with nor actively reinforced anything the ADSD has wanted to do up to this time.

Chief of Medical Staff (CMS)

A married male in his early forties, the CMS is a newcomer to the hospital. He is very concerned about patient care and works long hours in the hospital making rounds and supervising the resident staff. The CMS is friendly with the ADSD, whom he knows as a fellow board member on a professional association. He often confides his frustrations about patient care to her and solicits her support in making organizational changes to improve patient care.

Background

Over the past few months there have been many complaints about nursing care from patients and physicians. The usual lack of supplies and poor staffing seem to have gotten even worse. The staff nurses have been to the DON to complain about their problems but have met with passivity. The RNs are now talking about organizing.

The ADSD is trying to get support for a training program for intensive care nurses, many of whom are inexperienced in intensive care nursing. The DON is being rather evasive about this proposal even though she agrees it is important. The ADSD is also upset about a recent incident in the operating room. According to those involved, the operating room supervisor suspected that she had some drug users among her staff. She also suspected these same individuals of pilfering and tampering with narcotics in the recovery room. The supervisor wanted to investigate further in order to correct the problem and elicited the ADSD's support in the investigation. The DON told the two of them to keep hands off, as it was too risky and might be perceived as harassment. The operating room supervisor persisted in her attempts to get data and was fired by the DON.

THE INCIDENT

The CMS, fed up with the poor nursing care, has had his residents document multiple examples of orders that were never carried out, delayed in implementation, or carried out incorrectly. Although some of the examples are rather petty, most of them are serious and are indicative of unsafe nursing care. In several cases patients sustained complications and had to stay in the hospital longer than would have ordinarily been necessary.

The CMS has presented these examples to the DON and asked her to do something about correcting the problems. The DON's response was to call a meeting of the supervisors and criticize them. No interventions or solutions to the problems have been planned or attempted.

The CMS, seeing no improvement or attempts at change, went to the HA with the documentation and demanded that the DON be discharged. Nothing happened--no action was taken by the HA.

EPILOGUE

Six months after the incident the ADSD resigned in frustration and was not replaced.

Twelve months after the incident the CMS resigned in frustration.

Three months later both staff development instructors who reported directly to the DON resigned.

Four years after the incident the hospital merged with another similar institution in the city, and the DON was appointed as nursing director for both hospitals.

Questions

1. Explain the DON's apparent organization success.
2. Where did the CMS and the ADSD go wrong?

case study 4

A major turnaround

Setting

A 250-bed, privately owned intermediate care facility is the setting for this case. The facility is located in the heart of a large city, in close proximity to a university medical center. The facility is about 18 years old and since its beginning has been beset with multiple fiscal problems.

The present owner, a one-man corporation, is the fourth owner. The building itself is owned by a two-man investor corporation from another state and is leased by the present owner of the facility. The present owner served as a consultant to the previous owners and two years ago bought the license to operate and lease the facility.

Approximately 80% of the patients in the facility are Medicaid, 15% Medicare, and 5% private-pay. Eighty percent of the patients are black, as are 95% of the staff. There are about 80 full-time personnel in the nursing department, and they provide 1.9 hours of patient care per day.

External Environment

The facility is located in a renovated area of the city that is both residential, with many long-term residents, and commercial; it is known as an affluent area.

There are other long-term care facilities in the city, all of which are competitors. This facility has had a bad reputation for the past 15 or 16 years. Its fiscal problems are well known;

it is also known for its poor care and is not considered a good place to work.

Internal Environment

The major norms in the organization are violence and do-nothingness. There are often physical fights among staff. A previous Director of Nursing was beaten up by staff. An attendant who was locked out of the building at night (he was several hours late for work and the doors are kept locked at night) used a sawed-off shotgun to open the door. Violence is tolerated and few staff are fired for their involvement in fights and violence.

Raises are automatic regardless of whether one performs on the job or not. The employee with the longest service has been with the organization for only seven years. Working conditions are poor and most people are there because jobs are hard to find elsewhere. In essence, they are putting in time. In fact, shortly after the new Director of Nursing came, she made rounds on the night shift (the first ever to make rounds on any shift other than days), and she found half the night shift personnel drunk.

The nonprofessional personnel are unionized, but they have a very weak union. Three months after their contract expired, the union threatened to strike. They did not strike and signed a new weak contract six months after the old one had expired.

Principal Players and Supporting Characters

Owner/Administrator

The owner, a good-looking, 37-year-old, married male, is described as a silver-tongued, smooth-talking guy with a lot of charisma. Everyone idolizes him. He has his PhD in divinity with a minor in business administration. He was known to have saved several other nursing homes from worse situations than the present one, so his taking over this facility was viewed with great anticipation. By his own admission, though, he was "into making a lot of money." Although he was crisis oriented and did well in times of crisis, he could not exert leadership for the future; he could not set direction.

When he bought the nursing home in 1981 the owner hired a female administrator, with little management experience, and a Director of Nursing, diploma-prepared and also with little administrative experience or skill. He left the operation of the nursing home to the administrator and the Director of Nursing, visiting the facility only occasionally. In 1983, because the nursing home was in trouble, he fired the Director of Nursing and subsequently hired the current one. He quickly became quite attracted to the new Director of Nursing, fired the administrator, and assumed the position of administrator himself. Thereafter he was at the nursing home almost daily, although he lived 150 miles away in another state.

Director of Nursing (DON)

The current DON was hired by the owner in 1983. She is a 43-year-old, master's-prepared nurse who has seven years experience in gerontology. Her experience includes both clinical and management responsibilities. She had previously "set up" a nursing home--in essence started it from scratch--and had trained all the staff that she had employed. The care at her previous facility was known for its high quality, and the nursing home was known as a good place to work. Because there was potential for the nursing home to become affiliated with the nearby university, the DON wanted an appointment with the school of nursing. Therefore, the school of nursing hired the DON, and the owner contracted with the school for her services. She did not, at this time, carry any school or teaching responsibilities.

Medical Director

The Medical Director is a young, progressive physician from the university who has hopes of developing a "teaching nursing home'' here. He is the attending physician for the majority of patients at the facility, although a few patients have private attendings. He is a dreamer with great ideas who loves gerontology. He is a very caring physician. He decided that he wanted to have a nurse practitioner on his team, and in late 1982 he hired one who worked with him in the nursing home.

Nurse Practitioner (NP)

The NP is a geriatric nurse practitioner who shares many of the Medical Director's goals and dreams. She has had many years' experience in gerontology. She also has hopes of developing a ``teaching nursing home,'' one that would demonstrate the value of the NP/physician team.

Background

In January 1983, state surveyors visited the nursing home for review of the facility's compliance with state standards. Their report was reviewed by federal investigators, who did not agree with the report. In February 1983, federal investigators arrived at the nursing home to conduct a one-week survey. (In essence, they were checking on the state surveyors.) The arrival of the federal investigative team coincided with the arrival of the new DON.

The federal investigative team gave the nursing home 60-day notice to shape up; otherwise they would revoke the facility's license and close the nursing home. They charged the state surveyors with covering up. Thirty pages of citations and deficiencies were noted; the majority of them were in nursing. The new DON had her work cut out for her.

The DON started many new programs. For example, she provided orientation and in-service programs which had never been provided before. She enlisted the support and help of the NP, who taught staff on a one-to-one basis. Very quickly, the staff responded to this attention and teaching, and clinical nursing care improved. The DON instituted narcotic counts; they had never been done before. There was absolutely no documentation; she taught staff how and what to document. There had been a high medication error rate; she replaced all the certified medical technicians, who were in charge positions, with LPNs. The medication error rate dropped.

The DON also hired an Assistant Director, a young, black nurse, the only black in the administrative hierarchy. The Assistant Director did not want to take the position on a permanent basis, but agreed to be the acting Assistant Director. In her words, "I'm an Indian, not a chief." Although she had no management experience, she learned fast and was effective at operationalizing ideas.

In addition to focusing on patient care problems, the DON also paid attention to personnel problems and issues. She fired several staff who were incompetent and/or involved in violent incidents. She rewarded those who performed well. Staff began to tell her about how they were not being paid what they were supposed to be paid and about not being paid for overtime or given comp time. She corrected these problems and saw to it that staff were paid their due.

In May 1983, the federal investigative team returned to the nursing home. They noted "substantial improvement." In fact, they could hardly believe what they saw. The majority of the nursing deficiencies were gone. They specifically commended the new DON and also the owner, who had assumed the role of administrator.

THE INCIDENT

With the threat of license revocation and closure gone, the owner, the DON, the Medical Director, and the NP began planning for the future. They had passed their crisis and were now ready to develop a progressive, model program in long-term care for the elderly. The owner encouraged the staff to make "wish lists" and promised them everything they wanted.

In July 1983, the DON was asked to cut back on staff. The patient census was down and the owner said they would have to cut back temporarily. He said that soon, however, they would have more money, and he encouraged them to continue to plan for improvements. However, the DON did not cut back her staff because she already had only the minimum to cover all shifts.

In July, the owner hired one of the state surveyors as Assistant Administrator, and the DON, her Assistant Director, the NP, and the Medical Director continued to make improvements and to plan for the future despite limited resources. However, any recommendations for and attempts to change were constantly put off. By September and October, there were insufficient supplies for even the most basic of care.

In November, the staff requested an all-day meeting with the owner to look at where they had been and where they were going and to examine why they were backsliding. The owner continued with his promises and encouragement, even though he had shared with the DON his thoughts about selling. He had not shared this thought with anyone else. At the end of November, however, he shared with everyone his intent to sell. He also told them that their ambulatory service would be discontinued because the bill had not been paid for three months, drugs would no longer be provided by the university because that bill had not been paid for six months, and food delivery was threatened because that bill was also unpaid.

In mid-December, the DON was scheduled for a three-week vacation. Reluctant to leave because of all the turmoil and potential crises, she did so anyway because she had planned for a year for her trip out of the country.

Upon her return, she finds two new owners. The previous owner had sold out at a substantial profit. The new owners are people who can no longer get an operator's license in a neighboring state. The new owners were also the management group (by contract) for another private nursing home in the city and had been fired. Neither of these facts are encouraging to the DON.

The new owners approach the DON and ask her to get rid of all the RNs on her staff and to replace most of the LPNs with certified medical technicians.

QUESTIONS

1. What are the DON's options in this situation?
2. What is the probability of success for any of the identified options?

case study 5

Strained relationships

SETTING AND EXTERNAL ENVIRONMENT

This 125-bed long-term care residential center for mentally retarded well adults is located downtown in a large midwestern city. The facility opened in the 1960s and is part of a larger profit-making corporation that owns many nursing homes and one other residential home. The closest competing facility is located approximately 100 miles away. Most of the home's residents come from the immediate vicinity or from within a radius of 100 miles. Residents are referred primarily from community agencies and sheltered workshops. Funding for the center comes chiefly from Medicaid and private insurers, although few residents' fees are subsidized by their families' income.

The majority of the residents are permanent live-ins. Seventy-five percent go to work in sheltered workshops, stores, and factories in the immediate area. If a resident becomes acutely ill, he or she is referred to a community hospital for treatment. There is also a physician consultant who visits regularly once a week to make rounds. On-call medical emergency services are available at all times.

The agency occupies a three-story building that accommodates resident and staff housing as well as administrative offices. It is an old building and difficult to maintain in good repair. There is insufficient space for recreational activities. Privacy for both residents and staff is a problem. The residents share semiprivate sleeping accommodations and common bathroom facilities. There are a few private rooms, but these are given either to so-called problem residents or to those whose families pay their fees.

The agency's main goal is to find group home or adoption placement for its residents. Thus far, only about 20% of the residents have achieved this goal. The facility and its services have a good reputation in the community, and the facility is valued as a good placement by referral agencies.

Internal Environment

The organization is described as maintenance oriented with emphasis on preservation of the status quo. There have been few changes in this facility or at corporate headquarters over the years. The organizational structure is a traditional, centralized or vertically integrated organization with clear-cut lines of authority and responsibility. The organization culture is described as somewhat paternalistic but informal. First names are used by employees and management, at least within a work group. Employees are encouraged to bring suggestions and complaints to the administration's attention. Everyone knows everyone else, their jobs, and some of their personal business.

Turnover is low among staff even though salaries and benefits are not competitive with other health care agencies in the area. Nursing aides and therapy attendants are unionized; other employees are not. There is a sense of commitment to a mission of caring for the truly needy person. Residents are treated kindly and fairly. The administration has established an "employee of the month" recognition program that includes a cash bonus. This recognition program is a valued ritual of the organization.

The majority of residents in the home are Caucasian and Catholic. Management positions are all filled by Caucasians with the exception of one black female manager. The majority of staff are black. There are no overt or covert racial or ethnic problems between residents and employees or between staff and management.

Communication and information flow from the top down within the agency and from the corporation down to the agency. There are few "secrets," however, and information is usually freely given in exchanges between and among staff. Interdepartmental reports are held twice a day, once in the morning and once in the early afternoon. Dress code is informal with uniforms optional except for nursing aides. There are rules and policies for the safety and protection of residents, as well as the usual personnel policies, but there is a loose control of staff behavior. Few grievances are filed by union employees, and there has never been a strike threat by the union.

Promotion is usually from within. However, since there are so few jobs at the top, there are few promotional opportunities. Training for entry-level jobs is usually informal and on-the-job. Some formal orientation classes are held for nursing personnel, and monthly in-services are provided for everyone in direct patient care activities. These sessions are the responsibility of the Assistant Director of Nursing. Money is spent also on sending management people out to workshops and meetings.

The organization is small, with a total of 80 people employed at all levels. Of these, 45 are in the nursing department, 8 others are professional, and the remainder are nonprofessionals in support jobs, spread out among the other departments. The nursing department includes 4 RNs (2 full-time, 2 part-time); 8 LPNs all of whom have been in the organization for many years; 1 secretary; and 32 aides. Nursing covers all three shifts, the first starting at 6 a.m. and ending at 2 p.m. This very early starting time is meant to ensure that employed residents are ready to go out to their jobs in the community. Therapy sessions are scheduled around the residents' working hours.

The goals of the nursing department are prevention of illness and maintenance of health. First aid or short-term nonacute care also can be provided. Any serious or long-term acute illness is treated by referral to another facility. Long-standing contractual arrangements exist with hospitals and clinics in the city. Such referral arrangements are easily and quickly made through established contacts.

Principal Players and Supporting Characters

Administrator

The Administrator is a 32-year-old white male, married, who has worked at the facility for over 15 years. He started as a part-time attendant while attending college to become a social worker. He has worked his way up through the ranks, holding every management position except Director of Nursing. Described as an "old-school papa" type, he is considered an effective administrator and a good politician. His relationships with corporate personnel are positive. The staff in the resident facility respect his ability and like him as a person. He is willing to try almost anything if it has a good chance of working, and he is not a stickler for following the rules.

Director of Services

The Director of Services is a 28-year-old single female who has been with the agency approximately five years. She started as a recreational therapist, was promoted to Administrator of Recreational Therapy, and just recently (within eight months) was appointed to her present position. This position is a new one and the incumbent is the first person in the job. The corporation is interested in the possibility of using this organizational arrangement in other facilities and therefore is following closely how well this trial works.

The Director of Services has no formal management credentials and only an associate degree in her field. She is respected, however, for her knowledge about the mentally retarded and is considered an expert clinician. During her five years in the agency she has developed a strong personal and positive relationship with the Corporate Consultant for Non-

Nursing Activities. This consultant visits the facility on a regular basis.

The management style of the Director of Services is described as controlling and dictatorial.

Director of Nursing

The Director of Nursing is a 30-year-old single female graduate of a diploma school of nursing with a baccalaureate degree and a certificate in management. She has been with the agency and in the position for six months. Prior to taking this position she worked in several acute care facilities. She has had two years of management experience as an evening supervisor at a large metropolitan hospital and also some teaching experience. She left her previous job because she wanted better working hours. She is described as flexible and interested in improving coordination and teamwork among the therapeutic and professional services. She is intimidated by the Director of Services, whom she describes as a "put-down" person.

Administrator of Social Services

The Administrator of Social Services is a single, 31-year-old female who has been in the agency for one year. She supervises a second social worker who has been employed for two years. The Administrator of Social Services was formerly a peer to the Director of Services, who is now her boss.

Assistant Administrator

This other male manager is in his late 30s, married, and has been employed for four years. Like the administrator he has worked through the ranks and his formal credentials are minimal. He is responsible for nonprofessional services such as housekeeping, maintenance, and food service. He is well-respected and gets along well with his boss and the other managers.

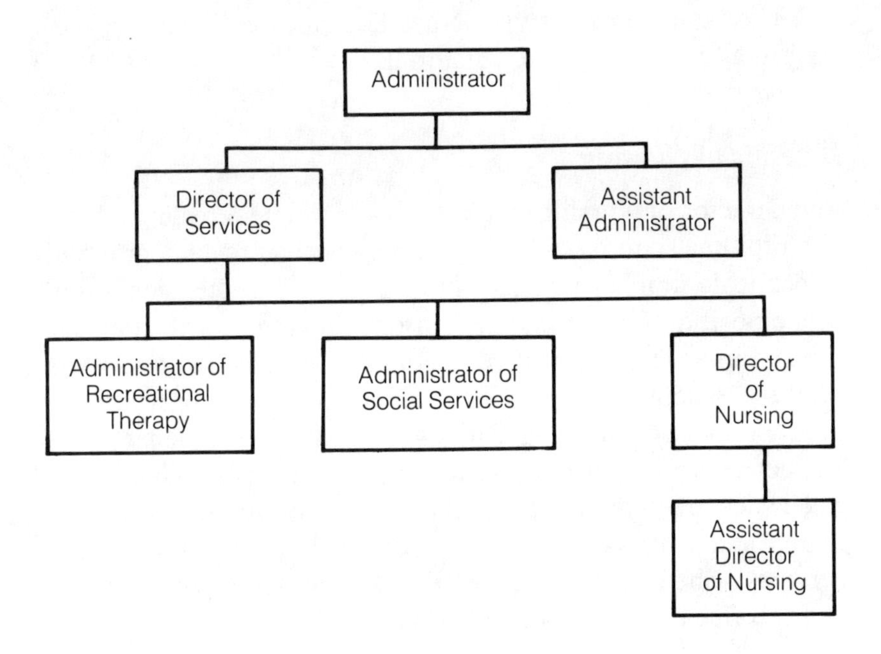

Administrator of Recreational Therapy

This position is held by a single, 24-year-old female who has been with the agency for two years. She supervises the two therapy aides, the total complement of the recreational therapy department. She maintains a cool and distant relationship with the Director of Services, who was her predecessor and continues to be her boss in this new organizational arrangement (see organizational chart).

Background

The Administrator has an office in a part of the building separate from the other management and administrative personnel. The Director of Nursing has a private office on the first floor. This office, a former resident room, was just converted and renovated recently. It is an attractive although small private space. This office is close to the therapy rooms and the shared office of the Administrators for Social Services and Recreational Therapy.

The Director of Services has an office on the third floor which she shares with the Associate Administrator. The Director of Services feels she should have a private office and wants the Director of Nursing to switch with her. Thus far, the Director of Nursing has made no move to do so, nor does she intend to do so.

The agency had two Directors of Nursing prior to the present incumbent's arrival. Both of these individuals are described as having been interested only in nursing matters and needs of residents. Neither worked as part of the interdisciplinary team, nor were they receptive to "organizational" needs. There was considerable conflict and much frustration expressed by other professionals, who strongly urged the Administrator to hire a nurse who would see the need for interdisciplinary effort. The present Director of Nursing understood this philosophy and desire when hired and has included as one of her departmental goals the need to improve teamwork with the other disciplines.

When the current Director of Nursing was interviewed by the Administrator only and agreed to take the position, she was shown both an organizational chart and a job description that indicated her position as reporting directly to the Administrator. In the interim between acceptance and coming on board, the organizational chart was changed to the current one illustrated. She was not informed of this change before coming, nor has her position description been altered. When the Director of Nursing became aware of the new organizational chart, she asked the Administrator if the Director of Services was now her boss. The Administrator declined to deal with the issue, merely stressing the need to "work together." Until the time of the incident to be described, he would not interfere in problems between the Director of Services and the Director of Nursing.

Relations between the Director of Services and the Director of Nursing have been strained the past four months. The Director of Nursing on one occasion suggested to the Director of Services that they meet to discuss their relationship problems but was rebuffed with the reply, "Just do it my way and we'll get along--I am the boss and can tell you what to do." The Director of Nursing has tried sharing her feelings of frustration as well as using problem-solving strategies. These two approaches have not been effective either. At the time of the incident to be described, the Director of Nursing has been using avoidance as a strategy to deal with the Director of Services. The Director of Nursing does have a corporate nursing consultant available to her, but thus far has not called upon her for assistance.

The Incident

One of the nursing department aides has a history of illness absences, usually on a weekend or before her days off. The Director of Nursing has spoken to the employee and advised her of the need to change this behavior. The employee did not change and was requested to bring a physician's verification note whenever she was absent because of illness. This procedure is seldom used in the agency but is described in the personnel policy manual and employee contract as a management prerogative when "deemed necessary." The employee, an old-timer who has "seen them come and seen them go," subsequently without telling either the Director of Nursing or the union delegate, took her case to the Director of Services, pleading unfairness and harassment.

The Director of Services received approval from the Administrator to countermand the order of the Director of Nursing. The Director of Nursing did not know of this action until the employee refused to bring in the physician's note after another absence and told the Director of Nursing, "The

Director of Services told me you had no right to ask me to bring a note."

Questions

1. What options does the Director of Nursing have for dealing with this situation?

2. Given the facts described, what are the risks of each option? What is the probability of success for each?

case study 6

The politics of illusion

Setting

This case study is set in a 500-bed voluntary acute care facility located in a traditional eastern environment. The agency, organized under local government control, is situated on a large tract of land within an urban setting. A private university hospital, an ambulatory care center, and a state psychiatric hospital are also located on the grounds. Established in the early 1900s, the agency now consists of the original building with some renovated sections and several brand-new floors. The majority of the new units are for intensive care and trauma patients. The main structure is a high-rise building consisting of eight floors. There are also a few separate, small structures housing administrative offices and support services.

One year before the incident related here, the governance structure of the agency was changed from governmental control to a complex administrative arrangement under the direction of three functional divisions. Control of these divisions is held by the private university, although the Board of Trustees continues the same as previously, with a mix of politicians, industry executives, and consumers.

The original mission of the hospital was to serve the poor and the destitute. In the past, the largest number of patients were to be found on the medical chronic care services, obstetrics, and trauma units. For years local politicians and would-be office seekers used the hospital as a focus for campaigning and vote-getting especially among the black minority who are served by the hospital and feel that care is substandard. Every year, additional public funds were allocated to make up the deficit between the $70 million budget and the income from Medicaid and Medicare payments. Occupancy, except in obstetrics, averaged only 70% of capacity, another negative financial impact factor.

The new mission is to continue to serve the poor and needy but also to attract middle-class paying patients. To this end, very intensive and expensive media and public relations campaigns have been mounted to increase occupancy to 90%. These campaigns emphasize a new image of quality care for all patients, rich or poor, black or white, and so on. Unfortunately, what is touted in the publicity is more illusion and hope than reality. As in the fable of the emperor's new clothes, however, drawing attention to this incongruence is neither highly desired nor greatly appreciated.

External Environment

The agency is located in an established, traditional community dominated by one or two main industries. These companies contribute heavily both to the tax base and to philanthropic causes. As a result, corporate executives expect to have considerable say about what goes on in the facilities to which they contribute.

The population of the community is predominantly white Protestant, with blacks being the primary minority group. The community is economically equally divided between rich and poor. The poor are equally divided between the ethnic majority and the minority black group.

Because of the presence of the large private university in the community there is also some division between town and gown factions. The city, one of the largest in the state, is also the county seat.

Internal Environment

Because of the change in governance, there are now two organizational cultures operating. The governance change brought in a new set of administrators who replaced all the former stakeholders, who were fired from their positions. There exists consequently both an old guard and a new guard, each trying to establish or maintain a set of values and norms that is opposite to the other's. Prior to the change, promotion was based on staying power in the organization. The new guard rewards and promotes those who support and promulgate the new image. Before the change, the old guard expected a hands-off, laissez-faire management style. Work got done, but productivity and quality were dependent on the informal leadership. Inappropriate behavior such as physical or verbal abuse toward patients and other staff was ignored or denied. Standards were loose and compliance with rules or policies was selective and inconsistent, even though there was a plethora of policies for every conceivable situation. Employees, particularly nonprofessionals, dressed casually in whatever attire suited them personally. The new guard has decided that there needed to be standards for conduct, including dress. After many long meetings of a committee composed of volunteer employees from all departments, a new dress code acceptable to the majority of employees was outlined. However, the new Hospital Administrator, a former military officer, vetoed this code and insisted on a more rigorous "spit-and-polish" attire for everyone. This reversal of the committee's work has become a cause celebre within the rank and file, who waste a great deal of time discussing and rehashing the issue.

On paper the organization is centralized, with everyone responsible in a line relationship to the Chief Executive Officer (see organizational chart). In reality, the chief executive position commands little authority, and everyone does pretty much as he or she pleases. Real power comes from political and university connections. Communication and directives flow from the top down but are selectively implemented. Conflict is con-

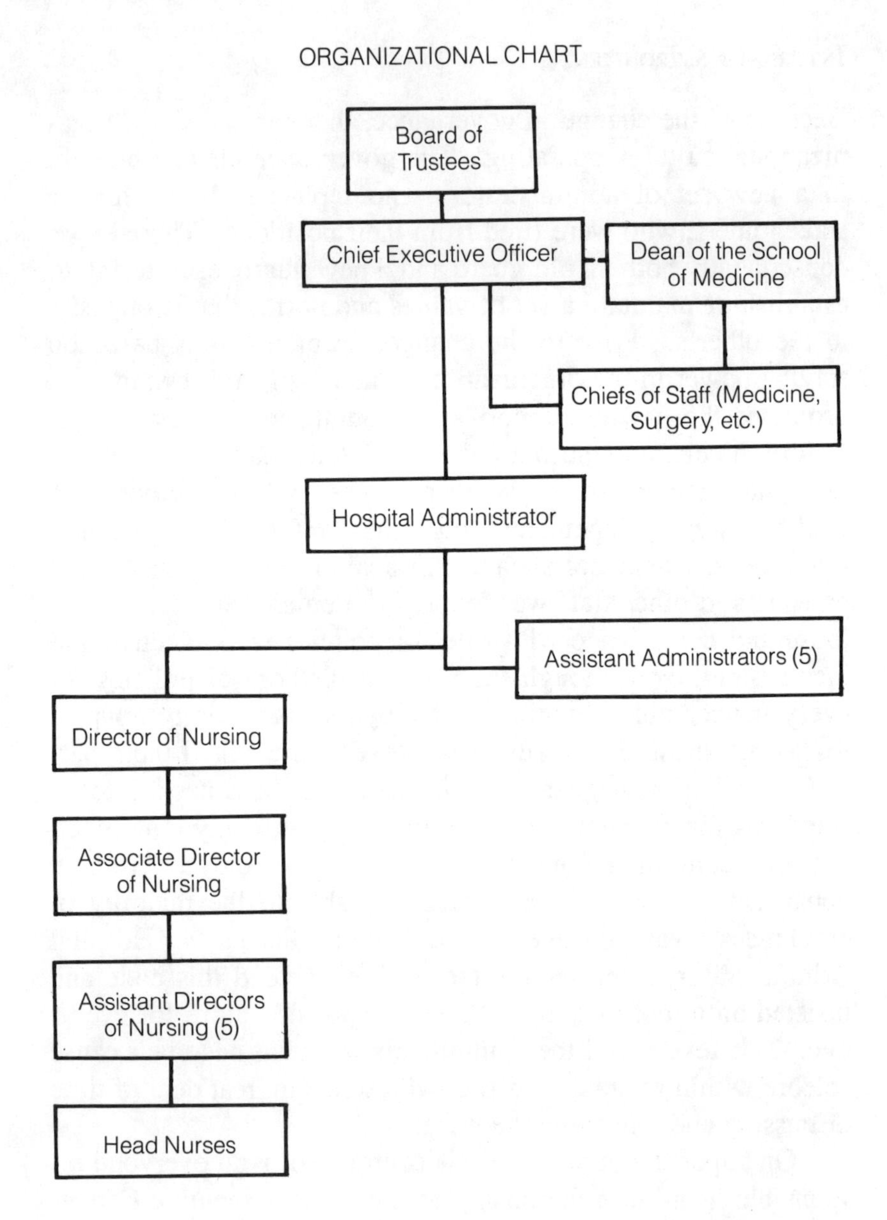
ORGANIZATIONAL CHART
Board of Trustees
Chief Executive Officer
Dean of the School of Medicine
Chiefs of Staff (Medicine, Surgery, etc.)
Hospital Administrator
Assistant Administrators (5)
Director of Nursing
Associate Director of Nursing
Assistant Directors of Nursing (5)
Head Nurses

stant but kept below the surface, with little direct confrontation between or among combatants. The new guard has established goals for high-quality care and performance, but there are few practical, concrete plans to achieve these goals.

The present personnel mix reinforces the two-culture reality. Budgeted positions exceed 2,000 full-time employees. Of these, 900 are allocated to the nursing department. Registered nurse and management staff are primarily white, Anglo-Saxon or Northern European Protestants. Nonprofessional staff are primarily black or other ethnic minorities. The nonprofessionals and a few remaining middle managers form the old guard. They resent and mistrust the new guard, considering them interlopers and opportunists.

Auxiliary nursing department employees are unionized but lack strong leadership. Government employees in this state are not allowed to strike. Consequently, salary and benefit are not competitive with private employers in the community. The grievance procedure is seldom used to force demands or concessions. In the old organization, nepotism was the norm. Thus many of the nonprofessional staff are related in one way or another.

Top management, before the change, treated employees somewhat paternalistically, although from a distance. Among the new guard empire building is extremely important and an overt criterion measure for success and achievement. External cosmetic projects such as new signs, planting of trees, and the latest equipment are funded without question. Money is freely spent, although it is unclear where it is coming from.

Principal Players and Supporting Characters

Chief of Medical Service (CMS)

The CMS is a male physician in his early 50s who has been in the organization since graduating from the university medical school. He has always believed that the hospital should be under university control and has an extreme vested interest in the new governance structure. Several years ago he had been appointed to the administrative post for the ambulatory care center, but was not a success in the position, even though he was responsible to the dean of the medical school at the university. His intentions are honorable. He is sincerely interested in quality patient care but tends to ignore practical realities. On paper he now reports to the CEO but views his relationship with the dean of the school of medicine as much more important and prestigious.

Chief Executive Officer (CEO)

The CEO, who has a joint appointment with the university, is a well-known physician-administrator in his early 50s. He has a national reputation, with connections to federal agencies and research foundations. He plays political games very effectively and maintains a cool, noninvolved stance. He came on board nine months before the Director of Nursing and was very instrumental in her decision to take the job. He has, in his nine months in the position, become very aware of the incongruence between public messages and reality. He is marking time until it is respectable to leave for another position.

Hospital Administrator (HA)

The HA is a charming, handsome, married man in his early 40s. He has had a successful 15-year career in the military and some additional civilian health care experience. This is his first position as an administrator in a large, complex agency. He is sincere in wanting to improve the quality of care, especially for the poor black patient population, but he is also realistic about the political nuances in the situation. As the only minority member in top management he is sensitive to the traditional values of the organization and the community. He has made many contacts with industry executives in the community and has involved himself and his family in community activities. He is very popular with the chiefs of services because he acknowledges their clinical expertise and does not presume to be their peer.

Director of Nursing (DON)

The DON is a single female in her mid-40s. A diploma graduate from a similar institution, she has had considerable administrative experience in nursing and holds a master's degree in nursing administration. She values being straightforward in her relationships with others and believes in calling a spade a spade. She admits to having a bit of a messiah complex but is sincere in wanting to improve the quality of care in the hospital. She is outspoken in her attempts to establish and maintain standards. A newcomer to the community, she has not involved herself yet in community affairs or established a network among other professionals or politicians.

Associate Director of Nursing (ADN)

The ADN is an attractive divorced woman in her late 30s. For several years she held the position of Research Assistant to the CMS. When the old guard was swept away in the governance change she was asked to be the Acting DON. She is well-liked and did not institute any major changes in the nursing service. She has no desire to be DON but is ambivalent in her support of the incumbent. For some reason she is out of favor with the HA, who wanted her terminated when the new DON arrived. There was no basis on which this could be done, however. The ADN continues to maintain her close ties with the CMS.

Assistant Administrators

There are five of these positions, all filled by white males in their early 30s, all with MBAs. None have any previous administrative experience, but all have served as consultants to health care agencies. All are very enthusiastic about the challenge of the situation and heartily endorse the public messages and new image.

BACKGROUND

In addition to the old-guard-new-guard dichotomy, a subculture exists within the nursing department representing former graduates of the hospital's still-existing diploma school. There is some talk of this school closing because of the university's recently established baccalaureate program in nursing. Such rumors stir the emotions and foment constant heated discussions. Before the organizational change, senior student nurses could work as charge nurses on evenings and nights, earning extra money and covering vacancies on shift. To the relief of some and the consternation of others, the DON on her arrival discontinued this practice.

The intensive care and trauma units, all new, are staffed primarily with RNs. The general units have 20% RNs only. On these units the aides, LPNs, and physicians had established an accommodating, democratic relationship reflected in a first-name basis and informal communication patterns. The new guard does not approve of this and prefers to reinforce the formal status differences. This has caused considerable resentment.

In the past, the nursing department focused on tasks rather than goals or objectives. The new guard emphasizes goal achievement, but in reality a tremendous amount of time is spent on personnel problems and issues. The new DON had to fire 47 people in her first month on the job because of absenteeism, unacceptable performance, or inappropriate behavior such as drunkenness. DON has also eliminated one level of management in the nursing department by having the head nurses report directly to their assistant directors. Most of the former supervisors have since left the agency. Of the five assistant directors, three are new guard and two old guard.

The DON's office, a newly renovated, attractive space, is adjacent to the HA's office. The DON has all the outward symbols of status, with appointments to the important committees. Most of the executive decisions are actually made, however, outside the formal structure through political and old-boy relationships.

Relationships among the players are complex. The CEO is supportive of the DON, but is one step removed and doesn't believe in undermining the HA's authority except when critical. The DON and the HA share common goals but do not agree on the means to the ends. The DON values direct confrontation on problem issues, an approach unacceptable to other administrators. As the only woman on the management team, she is perceived negatively because she does not support the public illusion.

Six months have passed since the DON took the position. Several incidents have occurred already that resulted in confrontation between the HA and the DON and required intervention by the CEO. The first took place just one month after the DON's arrival. It involved the lack of prepared RN staff for the trauma unit. The DON refused to open beds until there was adequate staffing. A great deal of media coverage had been given to this wonderful new unit and what a contribution it would be to the community. The HA and the surgical chief of staff wanted to open beds immediately. The CEO ultimately intervened to support the DON's position.

The second incident occurred three months later. In the middle of a heat wave the air conditioning broke down in the pediatric intensive care unit. The DON insisted that the children be moved immediately to another area of the hospital. The HA wanted to delay, believing the system could be brought back to working order quickly. The DON appealed to the CEO and the chief of pediatrics, both of whom supported her decision.

THE INCIDENT

It is two months after the pediatric incident. The DON has been approached by the Assistant Director for Obstetrical Nursing Services. On this extremely busy service, medical care is provided by resident physicians. These physicians have different values and backgrounds from most of the patients. The nursing staff are concerned about what they describe as poor medical and undignified treatment of these patients. No one has documented or substantiated any of these concerns, however. Residents in turn complain about the nurses' behavior toward them. The Chief of Obstetrical Services denies any problems with his residents and has considerable data to show improved morbidity and mortality. He does promise to talk to his group, however.

The nursing staff continue to complain and finally agree to meet with the DON and their assistant director to develop an action plan. After many meetings the staff group comes up with a plan for documentation and confrontation. Soon after this meeting, an incident occurs in the labor room involving a resident's unacceptable behavior toward an unwed teenage primipara. The nurse confronts him and documents the incident. He responds by "telling off" both the staff nurse and the evening charge nurse. Documentation of the incident is taken to the chief of service, who thanks them for the information. In the weeks following this incident the resident staff collectively begin to lodge formal complaints against the nursing care and incompetence of staff nurses. The best-prepared RNs on the staff are leaving because of what they describe as harassment. No one on the nursing staff is willing at this point to confront residents or document their unacceptable behavior.

QUESTIONS

1. What do you think will happen in the obstetrical service?

2. Forecast the immediate and long-range future of the principal players.

3. Defend your forecasts using both the facts given in the case and the concepts you have learned relating to organizational cultures.

4. What went wrong here?

case study 7

Vested interests

SETTING

This case takes place in a 250-bed acute care community hospital in a rural setting. The facility consists of three modern buildings which are all connected. These structures were built six years ago on the same site as the original hospital, which was built in the 1950s. The hospital is a voluntary, freestanding facility that provides service to the community as well as a large winter and summer tourist population.

Reimbursement for services is 55% federal Medicare, 10% state Medicaid, and 35% private insurers or self-pay. The agency's reputation in the community had deteriorated over the years to the point that it was on the brink of financial collapse. At this point, the Board, composed primarily of physicians and local tradespeople, decided to bring in a new Chief Executive Officer. He recruited and hired several new administrators, including the Director of Nursing. Seven years later, at the time of the incident to be related, the hospital has a 90% occupancy rate, is making a profit, and enjoys an excellent reputation in the community.

EXTERNAL ENVIRONMENT

The hospital is the only facility providing acute care services within a 40-mile radius of the community, a traditional one settled many years ago by farmers all belonging to a particular Protestant denomination and ethnic group. The community has since grown to include tradespeople and tourist business owners. The majority of old-timers are blue collar, and most belong to unions. Recently there has also been an influx of city folk who enjoy the benefits of country living but continue to work in the nearby cities. These people are considered outsiders and have little or no influence on political or community decisions. None of these outsiders are members of the hospital Board.

The Hospital Administrator was hired seven years ago, and his management team have developed and marketed a variety of outreach services, including executive health and fitness, screening and consumer education, and sports medicine programs. All of these efforts have been successful and are perceived as somewhat of a threat by the acute care facilities 40 miles distant.

Internal Environment

As a result of a gradual, planned change process taking place over the last seven years, a markedly different organizational culture exists in the organization even though the ethnic mix remains the same, primarily middle-European Protestant. A few of the old guard remain, but they are not influential in organizational decisions.

Prior to the planned change employees were formal in their relationships with one another, passive in regard to innovation, and were rewarded and promoted based on their community connections. There is now considerable interpersonal informality among staff with the exception of relations with physicians, who continue to maintain an aloof status within both the community and the hospital. Promotion is now based on merit and encouraged from within only when personnel are qualified. Employees, realizing that their jobs are not at risk as long as their performance is acceptable, have become supportive of the changes initiated.

Orientation, training, and development programs have been instituted by the new administration, who also continued the previously established support of outside educational opportunities. An attempt had been made to establish organizational rituals such as a Christmas party and softball team to bring employees closer socially, but staff resisted these efforts, stating they had families at home and did not need another one at work.

The organizational structure is very little changed from that in place seven years ago. The only major change was the addition of a position titled Associate Administrator. Three departments--pharmacy, physical therapy, and mental health--formerly reporting to the Hospital Administrator are now responsible to the Associate, whom the new Hospital Administrator recruited from outside the organization. Four other departments--nursing, personnel, emergency services, and finance--continue as before to report directly to the Hospital Administrator (see organizational chart).

Over the past seven years the management style has become more participative, with an open-door climate and two-way communication systems supported by most administrators. Although both goals and means are considered important, when a choice must be made goals or ends take precedence over means. Empire building is discouraged. Physicians, however, continue to see themselves as the power base and have formed group practices for almost every type of medical service. There are no resident or internship programs, but a number of physicians have hired their own physician's assistants. There are no nurse practitioners in the hospital nor are they looked upon favorably by physicians, who very effectively use their social connections and board positions to influence decisions made about hospital affairs.

Principal Players and Supporting Characters

Hospital Administrator (HA)

The HA is a married male in his late 40s who specifically moved to this community to take the position offered him by the board. He has considerable hospital management experience and is particularly expert in fiscal management. With a

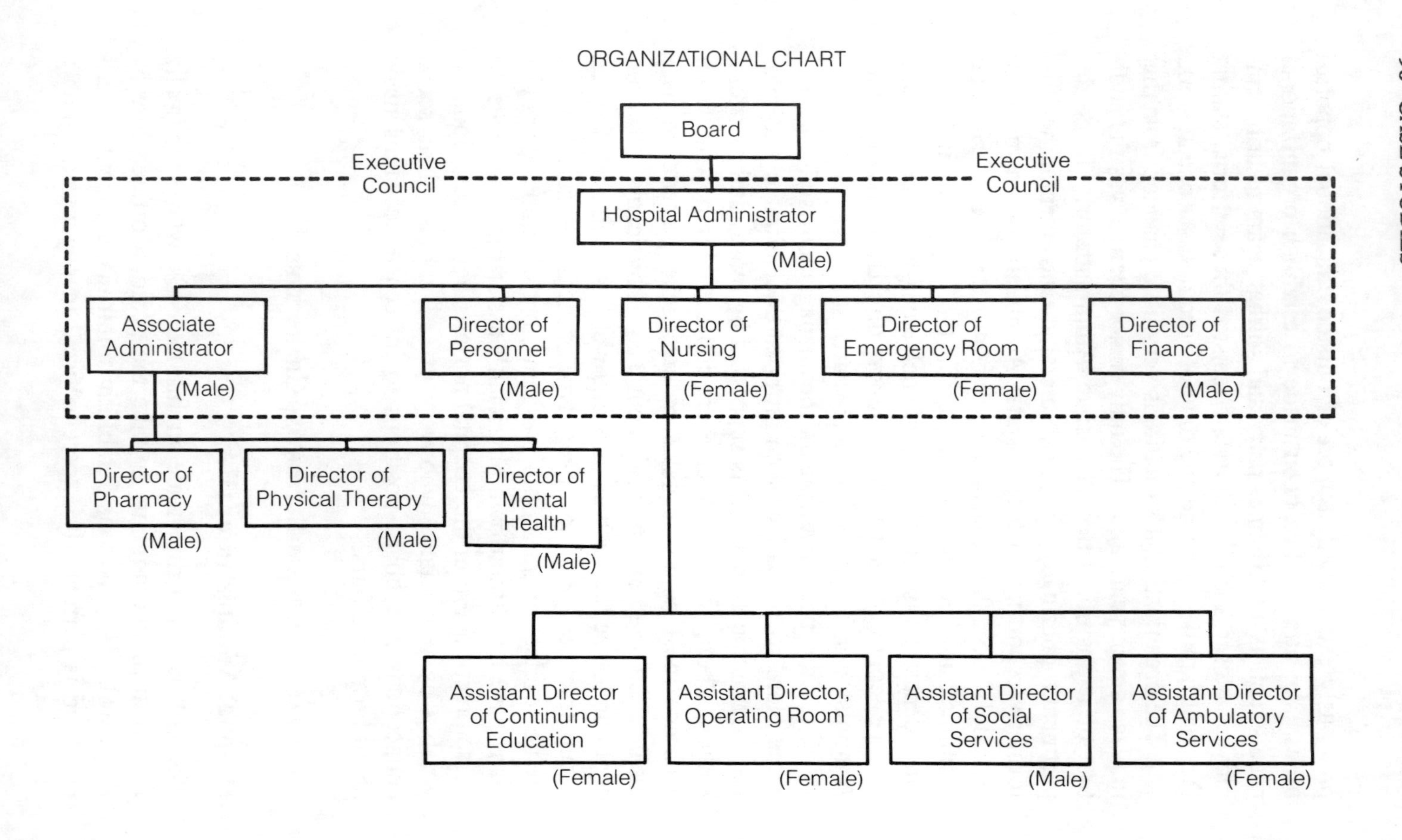
ORGANIZATIONAL CHART
Board
Executive Council
Executive Council
Hospital Administrator (Male)
Associate Administrator (Male)
Director of Personnel (Male)
Director of Nursing (Female)
Director of Emergency Room (Female)
Director of Finance (Male)
Director of Pharmacy (Male)
Director of Physical Therapy (Male)
Director of Mental Health (Male)
Assistant Director of Continuing Education (Female)
Assistant Director, Operating Room (Female)
Assistant Director of Social Services (Male)
Assistant Director of Ambulatory Services (Female)

previous background in counseling, he is thought to have excellent people skills and is described as smooth, articulate, and bright. He is well-liked by employees, who see him as friendly, visible, and approachable. His own administrative group perceives him as an effective manager. He is particularly supportive of nursing and enjoys an excellent relationship with his Director of Nursing.

Shortly after taking over, the HA perceived that the board, of which he is a member, was making decisions and taking actions that were rightfully the prerogative of management. The board acceded to the changes the HA demanded at the time, but there are some physician members who still feel that the board was stripped of its rightful power.

The HA has formed many contacts in the community and is active in service groups and community affairs. His wife and children also are active and visible in the community. The HA is, however, a member of a very different Protestant denomination and is still considered an outsider.

Director of Nursing (DON)

The DON, hired by the HA, is a single female with a master's degree and considerable nursing administrative experience. She had lived in the community two years prior to taking this position, but was working in a nearby city. She, like the HA, has become very active in the community, serving on several community agency boards. As a Catholic, she too is still considered an outsider. She has had several confrontations with physicians over the proper role of the nurse and what is acceptable and legal nursing practice. In every case, the DON was supported in her decisions by the HA. In addition to having a good relationship with the HA, the DON also has effective working relationships with the Director of Finance and the Director of Emergency Services, a nurse and the only other female executive in the hospital.

The DON is occasionally invited as a guest to meetings of the board, is a member of the Executive Council, and is a voting member of three medical board committees.

Staff Radiologist

The Staff Radiologist is a 40-year-old physician who was born and raised in the community. He is married to a nonworking diploma nurse who was on staff prior to the DON's arrival and remembers the old days. The Staff Radiologist has had several serious confrontations with the HA and the DON. The HA has supported the DON in her confrontations with the Staff Radiologist. The board initially supported the HA against the Staff Radiologist in their most serious confrontation, but then backed off and insisted on a compromise situation which satisfied neither the Staff Radiologist nor the HA.

Director of Mental Health

The Director of Mental Health is a 40-year-old male with a doctorate in psychology. At the time of the incident to be related, the RN staff in the mental health unit reported to him. He has developed many contacts with physicians and makes it his business to keep them informed of what is going on in all departments, particularly nursing. He is not a member of the Executive Council but is the Associate Administrator's appointed delegate when the Associate Administrator cannot attend executive meetings.

Director of Personnel

The Director of Personnel is a male in his late 50s who is described as incompetent but a nice fellow. His management style tends to be one of hopeful avoidance: he delays acting on problems hoping they will either go away or resolve themselves. He and the DON have had many confrontations in regard to the need for prompt response to complaints or concerns of nurses. The Director of Personnel is a good old boy and has many social and blood ties to nonphysician Board members.

Background

At the time of the incident the hospital is in excellent financial shape and continues to successfully diversify its outreach services. However, many physicians, initially supportive of the HA and his philosophy because of the hospital's severe financial problems, are now resentful of what they perceive as a coalition between administration and nursing against their interests and needs.

The nursing department includes almost half of the hospital's 800 employees. More than 50% of the nursing employees are RNs, with some LPNs, operating room technicians, and approximately 125 aides and clerks. The majority of RNs are diploma graduates. Baccalaureate nurses are being vigorously recruited, and a generous full-tuition benefit plan has been initiated to encourage further formal education. The DON has hired a master's-prepared educator (the only other master's-prepared nurse besides the DON) to head the department of education. This assistant director and the DON work very closely and are very supportive of one another.

Prior to the planned change, each nursing unit did what it thought best with few established standards or procedures. The DON and her assistant director have spent considerable effort and educational resources on developing practice standards and procedures.

Approximately half of the RN staff are described as being of the new breed, or more assertive, independent, and vocal, and champions of collective bargaining. Many of the other nurses are divorced single parents or contribute heavily to family income. These nurses need their jobs as a source of income and are concerned with salary and benefits more than career.

THE INCIDENT

For several years the state nurses' association has been attempting to organize the hospital's RNs. An attempt six years ago failed. However, the most recent attempt has been successful, a majority of RNs voting in June to accept the association as its collective bargaining agent. Contract negotiations began in September. The negotiation team consisted of 15 staff nurses, 2 union representatives, and 4 management representatives. After four months of bargaining, negotiations were declared to be at an impasse. A mediator was then brought into the situation.

During the negotiation period a group of physicians decided they would negotiate separately with the nurses. Although they had no authority to do so and were so advised by the legal department and management, they continued to meet with the nurses.

In February of the following year, eight months after the election, a contract offer was made by management. This offer was rejected and the nurses voted to go out on strike in March. The strike lasted for nine weeks. During this time occupancy was reduced to 50% and maintained by supervisory staff, LPNs, and the auxiliary. The Joint Commission on Accreditation of Hospitals and the state board of health visited the hospital during the strike. Both gave positive reports of nursing care and reaccredited the hospital. Also during the strike another union attempted to organize LPNs and operating room technicians. This attempt, however, was unsuccessful.

The strike was an extremely unpleasant experience for everyone. There was a great deal of verbal abuse and some physical violence directed at management personnel and their families. People in the community, particularly those associated with unions, supported the striking nurses and vilified management.

In the tenth week, a contract offer was accepted by the negotiation team and constituent members. This contract excluded a closed shop, gave one less holiday than was allowed before the union was organized and the same dollar salary increase as offered by management in February. As soon as the strike was over, physicians demanded that all beds be opened immediately. In the DON's perception this was an unreasonable request, and she refused to go along. The board also put pressure on the DON, but she was supported by the HA. Beds were opened gradually with complete occupancy achieved within three weeks.

In the weeks following the strike, the board appointed a committee to investigate its causes. This committee's report was not shared with the HA or the DON. The board, on the basis of the committee's recommendations, requested that the HA resign immediately, although he still had two months left on his contract. The HA resigned on the first of November. In January a multihospital corporation took over management of the hospital through a contractual arrangement with the board. In February the Associate Administrator resigned. In March a new Chief Executive Officer employed by the corporation arrived, and one week later he requested the resignation of the DON.

Poststrike Status

- The HA resigned and was replaced by a Chief Executive Officer salaried by the corporation.

- The Associate Administrator resigned and his post was eliminated.

- The DON resigned; her position was filled by an outsider hired by the new Chief Executive Officer.

- The Director of Mental Health remains in his position and reports to the Chief Executive Officer.

- The Staff Radiologist remains on board and is now both Chief of Medical Staff and head of the radiology group.

- The Director of Finance remains employed by the corporation.

- The Assistant Director of Social Services remains and reports directly to the Chief Executive Officer as a director.

- The Assistant Director of Continuing Education, Nursing resigned her post.

Questions

1. Explain the poststrike status of the various individuals and departments.

2. Could these outcomes have been prevented or changed? If so, how?

3. Forecast the future for the department of nursing and the nursing union.

case study 8

Intimidation and confrontation

Setting

This story takes place in an 800-bed facility located in a large midwestern city. An acute care facility over 100 years old, the facility occupies its original site and consists of several old buildings and one new one. All the buildings are connected and are undergoing constant renovation and repair. Because of the age of many of the buildings, maintenance and housekeeping are always problematic. Just keeping up with breakdowns and fumigations takes most of the available resources and time. Like the buildings, equipment is a mix of the oldest and the newest.

Ownership of the hospital has always been voluntary and nonprofit under the control of a religious order. The hospital's mission is to serve the sick poor, and the hospital has a past reputation for compassionate care of indigents, who make up approximately 20% of the inpatient population. Reimbursement is primarily from federal and state funds, with a small population of wealthy patients insured by private insurers.

External Environment

The hospital is located in one of the oldest sections of the city in a neighborhood that consists of a core of poor, mixed with middle- and upper-middle-class business people, and a huge colony of artists and artistic hopefuls. The latter group is in constant flux, coming and going as they lose hope or become successful. The middle- and upper-middle-class business group is very politically active in municipal affairs and tends to dominate the liberal minority party in the city. All ethnic and cultural groups are represented in the neighborhood, which encompasses an area of about 10 square blocks. Within this same area are three other competing hospitals. One, also under religious control, is much smaller and has been closed and revived within the past three years. The second is a large medical center with a different mission but offering the same types of services. The third is a medium-sized, private, not-for-profit hospital that three years ago merged organizationally with another, similar facility three miles away. All of the hospitals are holding their own with regard to share of the business, with the medical center slowly moving ahead of the others.

Internal Environment

In spite of the size and complexity of the institution, interpersonal relationships are quite informal. With the exception of private physicians and those belonging to the religious order, everyone is called by first name and all mingle freely in the hospital cafeteria. There are few rituals that everyone complies with or values, although there is considerable pride in the nonprofessional group about looking "professional," which usually means having a spotless uniform. Everyone complains about the dirty, broken-down appearance of many of the buildings and talks about how different it was in the old days. The housekeeping and maintenance departments, understaffed and stretched thin, are the objects of frequent complaints and are often scapegoated for all kinds of problems over which they have little or no control.

Promotions and rewards are based on loyalty, affiliation, and contacts. Although higher-level positions are filled both from the inside and the outside, over the past five years more and more top-level positions have been filled from the outside by strangers. Members of the religious order hold 10% of the management positions, including the top administrative post. With the exception of the heads of housekeeping and maintenance, all top managers are white. Within the hospital as a whole there is little ethnic or racial conflict, however, probably because of the long-standing diversity in the community.

The organizational culture is described as passive with a "*que sera, sera*" response to events. Maintaining the status quo is important, and any kind of change or innovation takes a long time to implement. Many in the organization feel that the hospital has changed dramatically over the last 30 years from a culture of dynamic leadership to one of acceptance and "what can you expect?"

There are lots of policies, but they are seldom followed, nor can they be found in writing. Everyone refers to the policy when defending or supporting a decision, but no one pays much attention or buys this rationale.

The organizational structure is a traditional, centralized hierarchy with information flowing from the top down (see organizational chart). Because there are lots of secrets, rumors and gossip are rampant. The culture is predominantly neither task nor people oriented. The party line is that personal needs should be sacrificed for the good of the patient, but that philosophy is not strongly reinforced or rewarded. There are no formal training or development programs outside of the nursing department, nor is much money spent on outside continuing education, again with the exception of nursing, which has committed considerable resources to staff development.

All employees including professional nurses, social workers, and pharmacists are organized under some collective bargaining unit. The only nonunionized personnel are managers and house staff physicians.

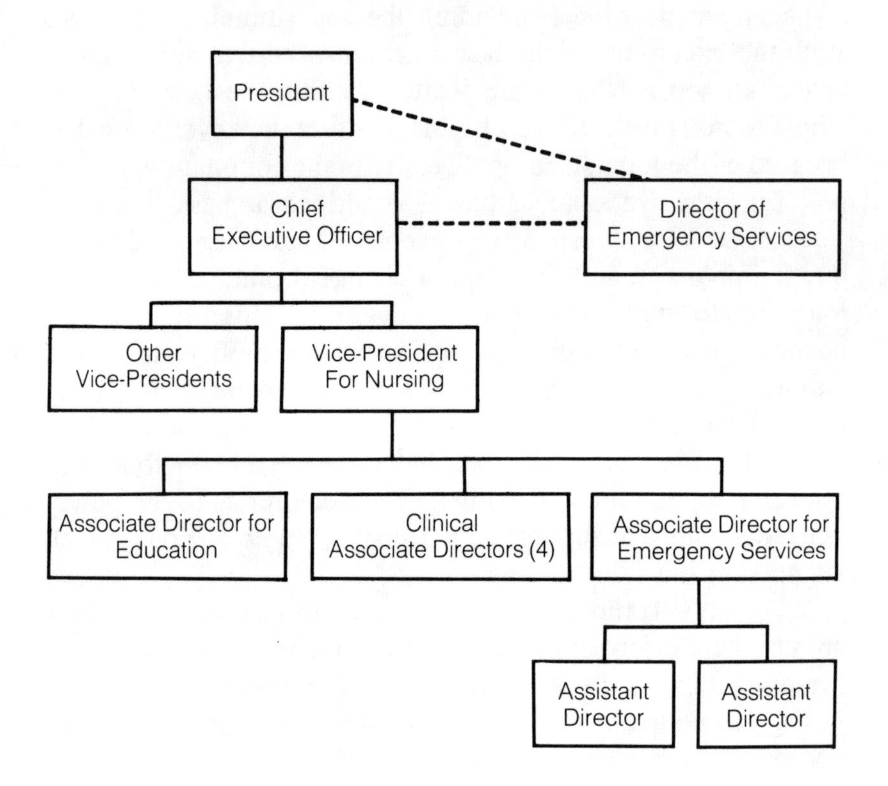

Principal Players and Supporting Characters

Chief Executive Officer (CEO)

The CEO is a married male in his mid-50s, holding a master's degree in public administration. He has been in this position for 18 months. He was recruited from outside the organization, and although he has no previous hospital administrative experience, he has held several important high-level governmental positions. He is described as attractive, entertaining, likeable, and very political. He has made himself very visible, mixing with the troops and using his excellent interpersonal skills. He is the first lay CEO in the hospital and was denied his request to have the title of President. The CEO brought in the Vice-President for Nursing (female) and several other new vice-presidents, all of whom are males, new to hospital administration, and lacking in formal educational credentials. They were recruited and hired primarily because of their connection and friendship with the CEO.

Vice-President for Nursing (VPN)

The VPN is a married female in her early 40s, new to the organization, who has been in the job for six months. She replaced an individual who was laissez-faire in her management style and rarely supportive of nurses and nursing issues. The VPN, hired because she had the right image and the right credentials, spent her first few months in the job being overtly supportive of nursing and very visible on all units and shifts.

The VPN reports directly to the CEO. She brought in several new associate directors and removed the one previous associate director, for whom a place was found elsewhere in the organization because of her seniority and loyalty to the institution.

The VPN, master's prepared, is described as controlling, autocratic, and cold. She has gained a reputation among her own managers of being a put-down person. Several members of the hospital management team also believe they have been publicly humiliated by her and as a result bear strong negative feelings toward her.

Director of Emergency Services (DES)

The DES is a male physician in his early 50s who has been in the organization for over 15 years. He does not practice clinically but has excellent political skills. He is described as ingratiating and superficially friendly. He enjoys considerable support from the President of the organization, possibly because he brings in a lot of money from federal grants and projects. The

DES also has numerous connections in high places in the federal government and in accrediting agencies. It is not clear to whom he reports in the organization. The DES and the VPN do not get along well and are described by others as adversaries.

Associate Director of Nursing for Emergency Services (ADES)

The ADES is a female in her late 50s and a member of the religious order. She is a graduate of the hospital's now-closed school of nursing and has spent 20 years in the hospital, seven of those years in her current position. She is described as serious with no sense of humor and somewhat devious. Handpicked for the job by the DES she has always reported to the Director of Nursing. Prior to the VPN's coming, however, there was little accountability expected of her from the Director of Nursing. Although the ADES has a smaller area and fewer staff than the other associate directors of nursing, she has two assistant directors reporting to her; the other associates have none. The ADES also was able to institute a new position of nurse practitioner at the same time other departments were having positions eliminated or frozen.

Background

Since the hiring of the new lay CEO and his management team, there have been a number of financial crises within the organization. Several middle managers have resigned or been terminated. In the nursing department there are daily staffing crises because of a general nursing shortage in the city. Staff nurses, who represent 60% of the 1,000 positions allocated to nursing, are equally divided between novices, or those with less than one year's experience, and old-timers. The organization structure in the nursing department follows the centralized pattern of the total organization. Of the management team 65% are old guard and 35% newcomers. The nursing offices are located in the same general area as those of the CEO and the President, but are smaller than and separate from the other vice-presidents' offices, which are located in a separate building.

Functional nursing is practiced on most units with an emphasis on safe technical care. The nursing department once had a national reputation but is now considered behind the times by outsiders. Because of the chronic shortage, supplementary staffing is a way of life, particularly on nights and weekends.

The Incident

Several weeks ago, the DES renewed a campaign, temporarily suspended when the VPN was hired, to have all employees in the emergency services unit, including the ADES and the RNs, report directly to him. The VPN responds that it is unacceptable that RNs should report outside the nursing department, even though operating room and mental health unit nurses are not under the control of the nursing department. The CEO, asked to arbitrate the conflict, suggests a compromise with a dual reporting responsibility for the ADES and has a new position description written for the job. The VPN, in a discussion with the DES and the CEO in the latter's office, maintains she cannot accept the compromise and walks out of the meeting.

The CEO, after waiting 12 hours to hear something from the VPN, assumes she has resigned and sends a telegram to her home accepting her resignation. The staff nurses, hearing of the incident through rumor and gossip, rally to the support of VPN, whom they feel has been treated badly. This staff nurse group contacts the VPN, who suggests they initiate a letter-writing campaign to the Board of Directors. The staff group intimates that unless the VPN is reinstated they will picket and perhaps even strike. The CEO agrees to meet with the staff in a mass meeting in which he states he will not take the VPN back. He is supported in his stand by his administrative team of vice-presidents. The CEO is put under considerable pressure by the Board, who do not wish to see picketing of the hospital. Two weeks after walking out of the meeting, the VPN contacts the CEO agreeing to the original compromise, and the CEO takes her back.

Questions

1. Forecast the short-term and long-term future for the VPN and the nursing department.
2. Was this incident a win or a loss for nursing?

case study 9

Caught in a coup

Setting

A 30-year-old, 200-bed, acute care community hospital in a rural setting provides the setting for this case. The hospital, a voluntary, not-for-profit facility, retains the original four-story building, having added a connecting building which houses patients and patient services. The old building will be used after renovation for ambulatory and extended care services. There has been no change in ownership or hospital mission. Reimbursement sources are 30% Medicare, 20% Medicaid, and 50% private insurers and self-pay. The hospital has a good reputation for providing routine care and has little local competition, being the only community hospital in the area. Special needs, such as cardiovascular and neurological surgery and long-term rehabilitation, are met by referral and transfer to hospitals in the large cities 50 to 100 miles distant.

External Environment

The community is a very old, established, rural one with most of the citizens blue-collar and agricultural workers. There is no one predominant ethnic group, although most backgrounds are European. Few representatives of racial or religious minorities live in the community. People tend to stay in the community, with few newcomers choosing to live there and few old-timers moving out. People don't go into the big city much, even for shopping or entertainment. It is a stable, conservative, traditional community. There is no major industry except for a large psychiatric facility that serves as one of the few remaining inpatient institutions in the state. The patients from this facility are often brought to the hospital for acute care services or follow-up care.

Most of the people in the community are poor or lower-middle-class. There are few cultural resources in the community but a great many local bars and corner taverns. Drinking and visiting are popular pastimes, as is drag racing down Main Street. The latter pastime results in a great many vehicular accidents and deaths. As a result the hospital has a very busy emergency room, particularly on the 11 P.M. to 7 A.M. shift.

Internal Environment

Because everyone knows everyone else and may even be related, informality reigns in the hospital with the exception of interpersonal relationships with physicians, who are always addressed as "Doctor." The physicians are very powerful. They demand and get constant respect and obedience.

Until the arrival of the new Hospital Administrator, rewards were given for maintaining the status quo, for supporting the organization, and for longevity. Everyone knows everyone else's business, including who is sleeping with whom, and gossiping is one of the chief entertainments. Everyone is friendly, and there are few status differences except, as already indicated, for physicians who enjoy an elite status. Everyone, except physicians, eats and socializes together outside the hospital. The June picnic and the Twenty-Year Club annual dinner are established hospital rituals that require attendance and participation.

Promotion has always been from within the ranks, and few managers have any formal educational credentials. Informal communication systems are used to get what is wanted, and there is rarely any direct confrontation between or among individuals with conflicting needs or interests. There have been few changes within the last 25 years except for the renovation of the physical plant.

There is a strict formal dress code for employees, and everyone is expected to be tidy, clean, and in complete uniform. All nurses, including the director and supervisors, wear full uniform including caps. Non-nursing managers, all male, are expected to wear ties and jackets. There are very few other formal rules. Most employees know what their jobs entail and perform appropriately. Supervisors are more like peers, often working at the same tasks with their subordinates. Supervisors have a difficult time handling problem employees because of lack of experience and guidelines.

The organizational structure is centralized with all department heads reporting directly to the Hospital Administrator. Traditional titles of Administrator, Assistant Administrator, and the like are used, and the chain of command is well understood by employees. Communication has always been open with few secrets or rumors before the change in administration. Until the arrival of the new Administrator, no one had a fancy office or a reserved parking space, except the physicians who have their own lot. Office furniture was old, often mismatched, and comfortable. The administrative offices were located in the basement along with the food service and the laundry. The new Administrator has had his office moved to an elegant, new, professionally decorated space off the lobby on the first floor. He also has a reserved parking space.

Previously there were few formal systems for evaluation of performance or outcomes, little quality control, and no formal training or development. There are no unions even though salaries are uniformly low. Merit increases or bonuses are not given, only across-the-board increments that everyone receives once a year. Employees are people rather than task oriented; means are more important than ends; and being politically savvy is more important than efficiency or performance.

The medical board is extremely strong with a number of physicians also serving as voting members of the Board of Trustees.

PRINCIPAL PLAYERS AND SUPPORTING CHARACTERS

Hospital Administrator

The Hospital Administrator is a big city-born and raised male in his middle 30s, married to a highly educated professional nurse who wants to continue working but is finding it difficult to get a job in the community. The Hospital Administrator is also highly educated, has spent several years in academia, and has published extensively on hospital administration. A member of a religious minority, he is described as brusque, sharp, and theoretical. He has high expectations for himself and others and little tolerance or patience with those managers who are not very bright or fiscally sophisticated. He was hired approximately one year ago by the Board to change the status quo and bring the hospital up to date. The Hospital Administrator is systems oriented and believes in long-range and strategic planning within a formal process. Acknowledged as technically competent, he is not very political and faces conflict with confrontation. Several months after he was hired, he employed a nurse consultant to work with him to reorganize the department of nursing, a task he feels has high priority.

Assistant Administrator for Personnel and Purchasing

The Assistant Administrator for Personnel and Purchasing, a single male in his 40s with no formal management or educational credentials, has come up through the ranks. He has close ties with the Assistant Director of Nursing and several members of the Board. He is very low-key but highly political and is well-liked by physicians, whom he purposely cultivates. Having lived in the community all his life, he knows everyone, their values, and the community norms. He was previously also responsible for financial affairs, a responsibility now assumed by the Hospital Administrator. The Hospital Administrator has recently teased the Assistant Administrator for Personnel and Purchasing in executive committee meetings about a physical deformity--something that has never openly been acknowledged or referred to by him or anyone else.

Director of Nursing

The Director of Nursing is a widowed female in her middle 50s with grown children living in another part of the country. She has a master's degree in nursing administration and previous experience as a nurse administrator, but most recently she has served on the faculty in a school of nursing. She moved here just three months ago after having been hired by the Hospital Administrator. Never having lived in a rural community before, she is experiencing difficulty adjusting to a different lifestyle and set of values. She has not yet had time to establish herself in any way in the community. The Director of Nursing agrees strongly with the Hospital Administrator's goals and objectives for the nursing department and is looking forward to a reorganization. She has not yet made any additional changes but wants to establish more professional standards of care and a performance evaluation system. Described as hard-working but disorganized, she is still trying to sort out relationships and hidden agendas. She has spent time on every shift and made considerable effort to meet all nursing staff. She also makes unit rounds every day, visiting patients with the head nurses.

Assistant Director of Nursing

The Assistant Director of Nursing is a married local woman in her early 40s who has come up through the ranks. She is a diploma graduate with no additional formal educational credentials. She had been the Director of Nursing for several years prior to the Hospital Administrator's arrival on the scene. Described as a very pleasant person, she is very popular with most physicians, to whom she caters. She is friendly with the other managers, especially the Assistant Administrator for

Personnel and Purchasing. Her management style is nonconfrontational and by exception; that is, she only deals with problems after they have been identified by others. She manages primarily from the office although she does know everyone's name and personal history. Thus far she has taken a neutral posture with the Director of Nursing, neither undermining her nor vigorously supporting her. The Assistant Director of Nursing has provided information on request and has volunteered to be responsible for staffing.

Background

One year ago several nonphysician members of the Board, described as movers and shakers, led a campaign to shape up the hospital and change its image. Since the then-Hospital Administrator was retiring, the time was right to get a sharp, new fellow in who could orchestrate the desired change. The new Hospital Administrator was subsequently hired and began to institute the needed changes. He shifted administrative responsibilities and instituted new systems and procedures. One assistant administrator was terminated and his duties were redistributed. As already indicated, the Hospital Administrator took over fiscal management from the Assistant Administrator for Personnel and Purchasing. The Hospital Administrator also instituted a long-range planning committee that included himself as chairman, the two Board members who encouraged his appointment, several carefully chosen physicians, and several other managers including the Director of Nursing and the Assistant Administrator for Personnel and Purchasing. All new programs and requests for capital equipment must be submitted to this committee with a detailed proposal including a financial plan. The committee must approve the proposals before implementation. As a result, several pet programs and equipment requests of physicians have been denied.

Shortly after his appointment the Hospital Administrator informed the Assistant Director of Nursing, who then was

Director of Nursing, that she was not his choice as Director of Nursing since she was neither qualified to implement the new responsibilities of the job nor able, in his opinion, to effectively achieve the desired goals and objectives. Rather than terminate her or ask for her resignation he made her the Acting Director until he could hire the right person. In the interim the Hospital Administrator hired, on a two-year contract, a nurse consultant to start on the nursing department's reorganization. The consultant was to work through the Acting Director and concentrate on skill building for head nurses and supervisors. The consultant also developed a plan for orientation and staff development, a function that was practically nonexistent in the nursing department.

When the Hospital Administrator hired the present Director of Nursing it was with the understanding that she use the Acting Director as an assistant for three months, after which time the Assistant Director of Nursing was to be evaluated based on a set of specific objectives and criteria. If the Assistant Director of Nursing did not meet the criteria, she was to be terminated. The three months are just about over and the Assistant Director of Nursing has not measured up.

The Director of Nursing has found that the staff is kind to patients, and the nursing care is technically safe, although delivered in a functional system. There are few nurses with any academic credentials other than the associate degree in nursing. There are 100 full-time RNs, 40 to 50 LPNs, mostly on evenings and nights, and 60 to 70 aides. There is little staff development except in fire safety and cardiopulmonary resuscitation, and few people go to outside continuing education programs. Nurses' relationships with physicians are very formal and deferential. Until the Director of Nursing was appointed to her position, nursing had no determination in budget formulation but was told what they had to work with. All staff were hired by the previous director herself. The Director of Nursing believes head nurses should interview and hire their own staff, a goal she intends to implement with the consultant's help.

There are two factions within the nursing department, one for and one against the Assistant Director of Nursing. Those who support her think she has been treated very badly; those against her think she deserves what has happened to her because of her management by distance and exception.

The Hospital Administrator did not attend the June picnic, nor has he made many attempts to join the few community activities available. He and his wife go back to the city frequently for entertainment and culture. It is rumored through the grapevine that his wife has been very vocal about how backward and "hick" people are here.

The Incident

One week ago the Hospital Administrator went out of town to attend a hospital administrators' convention. During his absence a protest committee initiated by the Assistant Director of Nursing developed a petition which was circulated and signed at a mass meeting. The petition to remove the Hospital Administrator from his post was then delivered to a special Board meeting convened by several of the physician members who also signed the petition. The petition cited some of the Hospital Administrator's less popular decisions and general personal harassment.

The Assistant Administrator for Personnel and Purchasing neither signed the petition nor attended the meeting, although he knew about both. The Director of Nursing knew nothing about either the petition or the meeting and only found out through a telephone call from the Hospital Administrator. The Board, after bitter arguments between the movers and shakers and the physicians, agreed to let the Hospital Administrator go. On his return a shocked Hospital Administrator successfully pleaded his management decisions, but was strongly encouraged by the Board to resign, as they doubted how effective he could be in the future. The Assistant Administrator for Personnel and Purchasing was immediately promoted to

Hospital Administrator, and he promptly moved into the new, fancy office.

Questions

1. Speculate on the Director of Nursing's future in this situation.

2. What options does she have to exercise in the situation?

3. Could the Director of Nursing have done anything to prevent her being placed in this position? If so, what?

4. What do you think the nurse consultant should do about her two-year contract?

case study 10

Even heaven has problems

SETTING

The hospital in this case is licensed for 567 beds. For fiscal year 1982-83 it had 1,947 full-time employees, and a total of 2,432 employees. It is located in an urban area. Although the original hospital was built in the late 1800s, its present facility dates from the early 1900s. The older buildings have been completely renovated, and several new additions have been completed. Renovation and refurbishing of the hospital have been continuous, especially in the areas of neonatal intensive care, cardiac catheterization lab, day surgery, cardiac rehabilitation, and central service. The facilities appear modern, clean, and inviting. In addition, over the years the hospital has purposely acquired land surrounding the main site for possible future expansion. One three-acre parcel of land was converted to a 1,200-car parking area. Other land holdings in the adjacent neighborhood remain as single-family dwellings, an apartment building, and a funeral home. The homes and apartments are at various times utilized for storage or living quarters for medical residents and others affiliated with the hospital.

The hospital is a freestanding, not-for-profit institution and is part of a religious-affiliated health care system. There has been no change in ownership over the years, but there has been a recent corporate restructuring. Unlike the other hospitals within the affiliated system, this hospital serves patients needing tertiary care, particularly open heart surgery and neonatal intensive care. There is no psychiatric or chronic renal dialysis service, but the hospital does offer a hospice service. The hospital is well-known for its perinatal, cardiac, and oncology services.

The reimbursement mix for inpatients is 45% Medicare, 45% third-party carriers, 7% Medicaid, and 3% self-pay. Since one of the hospital's missions is service to the poor, it is attempting to attract more Medicaid or Medicaid-eligible patients.

External Environment

The hospital is located in an old, established community with strong pockets of ethnic groups. It is predominantly a blue-collar, moderate-income neighborhood in a city with diversified industries. It was once a neighborhood of well-to-do professionals, but like many urban neighborhoods it has undergone change through the years.

The fundamental soundness of the hospital is well-known and respected by professionals and the larger community. A recent marketing survey reported that its strong acceptance by patients and the community could support substantial growth in services.

Within a five-mile radius there are five other hospitals. In addition, there is competition with alternative delivery systems and urgent care centers. The hospital has the market lead in some specialties, especially obstetrics, but is in direct competition with three of the five other hospitals for acute and specialty services. In comparison with other, similar types of hospitals, the hospital is in a favorable competitive position from a cost standpoint.

The hospital has a strong areawide reputation. Only one other hospital is mentioned more often when people in the city are asked to name familiar hospitals. Patients give the hospital higher performance grades than other hospitals, and more area residents would choose it for hospitalization over other hospitals.

Internal Environment

During the past three years, the internal environment of the hospital has been undergoing change. For the first time in the history of the hospital, which recently celebrated its 100th anniversary, a member of the religious order is not the President. There have been frequent changes in the organization chart for both the hospital and the nursing organization.

The hospital is a teaching hospital affiliated with major universities in the area. The majority of personnel in leadership positions are prepared for their responsibilities with appropriate degrees and certification. The hospital has a commitment to education and has always been generous with monies spent on conferences and seminars outside the organization.

The mission statement of the religious order owning the hospital is the basis of the hospital's philosophy and long-range plan. The mission statement emphasizes care of the poor, and the philosophy highlights human and community development--goals needing clearer definition and institutionalization. There is a real focus on caring behaviors, and these are recognized and rewarded.

The organizational structure is intended to be decentralized with high performance expectations for managers (see organizational chart). There are still, however, some aspects of management that are very centralized; namely, recruitment and finance. The management style is participative, although there is no question that the President makes his intentions known. Expectations are set and performance is demanded.

The hospital has changed from a maternalistic environment to one in which people are treated as adults. Only maintenance and boiler room workers have a union. The organizational milieu is neither overly formal nor obviously casual. Many individuals are on a first-name basis. An important norm is that a professional image is conveyed at all times to the public.

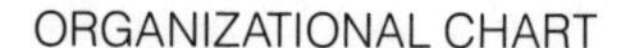

ORGANIZATIONAL CHART

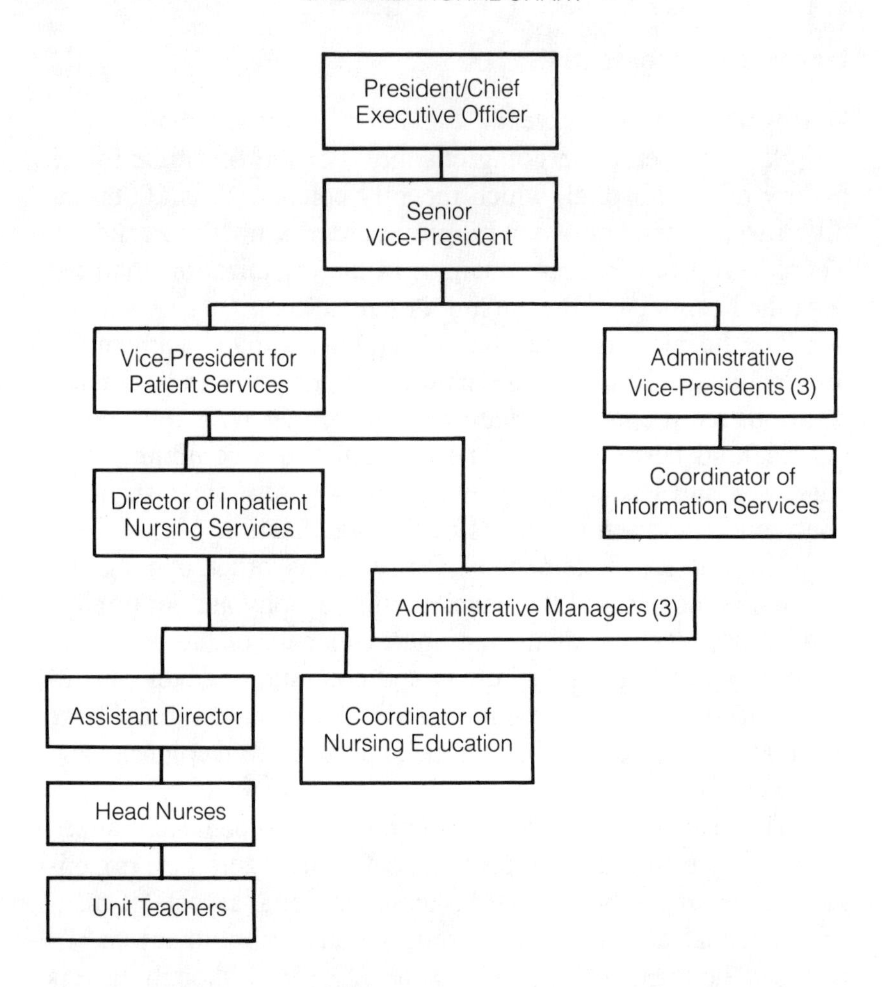

Nursing has prospered with the switch from a religious to a lay administration. Nursing's reputation, like that of the hospital, has always been outstanding. Despite their fine reputation, however, the administrative nursing quarters until recently were hard to find, being hidden away in a small, cramped corner. Likewise, nursing's previous involvement in upper-level management was not apparent. The new hospital President, however, has brought nursing out of the closet, and the nursing management team now enjoys modernly furnished and visible offices. The Vice-President for Nursing, the Director of Inpatient-Nursing Services, and other comparable nursing managers are active, full-fledged members of the executive team and important hospital committees. Nursing now has the visibility and recognition that it had earned and deserved over the past years.

Principal Players and Supporting Characters

President of the Hospital (HP)

The HP is a relatively young man, in his late 30s, who has developed high credibility with the staff. He is very forthright, direct, and honest. He is accessible and communicates well with all categories of workers. He is well respected within and outside of the organization and has surrounded himself with staff of comparable ability.

Vice President for Patient Services (VPPS)

The VPPS, also new to the organization, is a young master's-prepared nurse with considerable administrative experience. She is responsible for the ambulatory, surgical, and physical medicine and rehabilitation services as well as nursing services. She has appointed a Director of Inpatient Nursing Services and managers for the other services.

Director of Inpatient Nursing Services (DINS)

The DINS has been with the hospital a long time--over 25 years. She began working at the hospital after graduation and has worked her way up through the system, from staff nurse to head nurse to supervisor to associate director to her present position. She is master's prepared in nursing administration and has contributed greatly to the fine reputation nursing has in the larger community. She is a loyal and committed employee, and because of her tenure at the hospital she has a thorough understanding of the system, both historically and in its present context.

Coordinator of Information Services (CIS)

The CIS is an attractive female in her late 30s who has been in the organization approximately three years. She, like the other executives, was brought into the organization when the HP took over. She is an ambitious person, holding an MBA degree from a prestigious university. She is described as bright, cooperative, and on a "fast track." Although she reports to an administrative vice-president, she maintains warm, close relationships with the HP and is considered to be one of his favorites.

Background

At present, the nursing department is quite stable. The nursing department consists of a staff of approximately 1,000; 650 of these are RNs, with 565 of them in staff nurse positions. Staffing is very good; there are only nine open positions and these are primarily in the adult intensive care unit. Fifty percent of the staff nurses hold baccalaureates in nursing, nurse managers are all master's prepared in nursing administration, and the clinical specialists are master's prepared in their specialties. The nursing care is regarded with respect, internally and externally, and relations with physicians are generally positive. The nursing staff is not unionized, and there is no indication of such a movement.

Three years ago, however, the scenario was quite different. The community at large was experiencing an extreme shortage of nurses; internally, 25% of the budgeted RN positions were unfilled. At the same time, prior to the new lay administration, the hospital organization as well as the nursing department was centralized. In-service education was hospital-wide and reported to the human resources department, not the nursing department. The in-service education department consisted of a coordinator for education, three instructors, and a secretary. Because of the number of vacant positions, and consequently the number of orientations required for new RNs, LPNs, nursing assistants, and unit secretaries, the in-service instructors and coordinator were primarily involved with orientation programs in the classroom. Follow-up at the unit level for orientation and staff development activities was impossible for the already-overloaded in-service staff because of their classroom commitments. Furthermore, the in-service staff lacked some of the specialized clinical skills and knowledge necessary for putting together staff development programs. The assistant head nurses were supposed to provide follow-up orientation at the unit level and staff development programs. However, other responsibilities associated with the assistant head nurse position received priority. Consequently, unit orientation and staff development were left unattended.

As this situation became more and more intolerable, the lay administration came on board and decentralization began throughout the hospital. The DINS wanted to decentralize in-service education, but faced two problems: in-service education did not report to nursing but to human resources, and the hospital was under a mandate of "no new positions." The DINS was able to work with the Director of Human Resources, who agreed to a trial--an assistant head nurse position would be converted to a unit teacher position, and the unit teacher would report to the nursing department.

The DINS identified a head nurse/assistant head nurse pair who were willing to try the idea. Quite naturally, the pair were chosen because of the probability of their being successful. Quite conveniently also, the head nurse chosen was an informal leader of the head nurse group--if she thought an idea was good, other head nurses might also want to try it.

The trial was enormously successful, and other head nurses wanted unit teachers. They saw more value to the unit teacher position than the assistant head nurse position, particularly since they were moving into primary nursing and independent, autonomous professional practice. At the same time, the RN shortage ended and more RNs were being hired in place of nursing assistants and LPNs. A hierarchy at the unit level was no longer needed.

A year after the unit teacher trial, the assistant head nurse job classification was eliminated and converted to unit teacher positions. The in-service department now reported to the nursing department. The Coordinator of Nursing Education position and a one-half instructor position, for nonprofessional orientation, were retained. With a reduction of turnover, the job of the unit teachers and in-service department has become less one of orientation and more one of staff development.

The Situation

The decentralized system worked well and continues to work well, but, as with any system, it is not perfect. After a couple of years, several problems became apparent. These problems fall into four categories: patient teaching, unit secretaries, reporting relationships, and career ladders.

Patient Teaching

The unit teachers are responsible for assisting staff in patient teaching. However, formal teaching programs had been coordinated by the in-service department. There is a question of who is responsible for coordinating and teaching formal programs such as those for diabetic and ostomy care and the radical mastectomy and preoperative programs. There is also the question of who is responsible for gathering, reviewing, and keeping up-to-date all the patient teaching materials and aids. Some system for decentralizing these activities seems necessary to assure that they are efficiently accomplished.

The new prospective payment system may also affect patient teaching programs. Patients are now being admitted the day of surgery rather than the day before, making preoperative teaching difficult to provide. With reduced lengths of stay, there are also the questions of when patients will be ready for teaching and whether they will receive all that is required during a shorter hospital stay.

Unit Secretaries

The hospital has a progressive and coordinated automated data system, and the unit teachers do not feel qualified to orient and teach unit secretaries. The CIS is willing to orient and provide ongoing educational programs for unit secretaries, but in return wants the authority to assign, schedule, and evaluate unit secretaries in conjunction with the head nurse, to whom secretaries would still report.

Reporting Relationships

When the unit teacher classification was implemented, unit teachers reported to head nurses. After a short time, however, neither the unit teachers nor the head nurses liked this reporting relationship. Because the unit teachers work closely with head nurses, they both felt that they were really peers and thus collegiality between them was hampered because of the reporting relationship.

Career ladder

The nursing department has both a clinical ladder advancement system and a management advancement system. However, there is no mechanism for advancement for unit teachers--it is a dead-end job. The hospital and department are still under the mandate of ''no new positions,'' yet if the unit teacher role is to remain credible and viable, some system for advancement for unit teachers must be created.

Questions

1. Considering the past and present organizational norms and values and management style:

a. Will a dual reporting system with unit secretaries reporting to both the head nurse and the CIS work?

b. What other options could be considered?

c. What other reporting relationships for unit teachers would be effective and successful?

d. Identify possibilities for dealing with the unit teachers' lack of career mobility.

2. How might the questions identified in relation to patient teaching needs be answered?

case study 11

Comes the revolution

SETTING

This case takes place in a 900-bed hospital in the north-central part of the country. The hospital is located in an urban area and is affiliated with a prestigious medical school. One of the primary purposes of the hospital is to provide teaching opportunities for medical students, nursing students, residents, and interns. The hospital is physically connected with the schools and although not located in the center of the city, is easily reached by public transportation. The hospital, because of its affiliation with the medical school which has produced many "stars," attracts patients from all over the nation and even from other countries. The very latest in treatment and diagnosis is available in almost every medical discipline.

The site of the hospital is not the original one but has been in existence for 50 years. The several separated buildings are mostly old, although there are new units in each building. Space is always a problem and everyone competes for what is available. Major reconstruction is planned within the next five years. There is some ambivalence about this, as some of the open garden space will have to be sacrificed to accommodate the expected expansion.

The hospital has a long-standing tradition and reputation and has some of the most wealthy and illustrious citizens on its board. There is a high occupancy rate on almost every service. Elective private admissions sometimes have to wait three months before a bed is available. Ward services are also bursting at the seams, with frequent shuffling and temporary "boarding" of patients. Reimbursement is 50% private insurers, 35% Medicare, and 15% no-pay or welfare patients. In the past, large endowment funds made up for the charity care, a service that is considered vital to the teaching programs. This is no longer the case, however, and financial management is becoming a serious problem.

External Environment

The community in which the hospital is located was at one time a middle-class Anglo-Saxon neighborhood. It is now rundown and has a population primarily consisting of poor ethnic groups. Security is a constant problem. A high crime rate is a deterrent to recruitment of nurses, particularly for the night and evening shifts. The hospital has only limited parking space and some subsidized apartments, but these are insufficient for the demand.

The local residents resent the influence of the hospital in neighborhood affairs, believing that the hospital wants to take over real estate for its own purposes. In spite of these feelings, local residents use the emergency room and the outpatient clinics as their chief source of care, and prefer to be admitted to the hospital over any other choices.

In the new regime all vice-presidents and department heads are required to participate on community committees and be active in neighborhood government. This has met with mixed reactions. Some citizens see this involvement as positive interest and a desire to collaborate. Other residents perceive this activity as another attempt to "take over." These cynics support their perceptions with the fact that none of the administrators choose to live in the neighborhood.

Internal Environment: Before the Revolution

The hospital has always had a highly traditional and centralized organizational structure. A paternalistic administration assured employees that they would take care of them, and did. A clear caste system existed with physicians and the Chief Executive Officer being the brahmins. There was and still is a separate dining room for physicians, who were always addressed as "Doctor" except by the President, who is on a first-name basis. No space was set aside for nurse or employee lounges except in the locker rooms. Conference rooms were primarily for physicians and medical students, who had the prerogative of bumping anyone else who may schedule use of the space. In spite of the caste system, everyone was expected to treat one another like ladies and gentlemen; courtesy was expected and practiced. Rituals such as retirement dinners, an old-timers club, and Christmas dinner for patients and staff were religiously attended. Graduation from the medical or nursing programs was considered a must for organizational success. You earned your stripes through loyalty and belonging to the family; outsiders were few and not usually in positions of influence. It was considered an honor to work for the hospital, and employees were expected to obey the rules of the internal society.

Nurses were perceived as mothers or sisters, depending on age, length of service, and personality. Only white males have been allowed and continue to be administrators, except in nursing and social work where there are female administrators. Age rather than education or credentials was considered an asset; you learned your wisdom through the years with practice. Decision-making was concentrated at the top, but information was formally communicated through the ranks. Supervisors were expected to inform their personnel of the decisions for which they were then accountable.

Distribution of resources was unequal, with the teaching units getting the least or having to fight the hardest for supplies, equipment, and personnel. These units would have at the same time some of the oldest and most outmoded equipment and some of the newest. Supervisors and chief residents often joined forces to fight for what they believed was necessary for patient care. These coalitions established positive relationships for the future when the supervisor ultimately became the associate director and the chief resident became an attending physician or chief of the service. Although the teaching units had the fewest resources, they were considered the units with the best nurses, and for many years it was considered an accolade to be appointed head nurse or supervisor on one of the teaching units.

Relationships between and among groups were consistent with the established social order. Professionals always were one-up on nonprofessionals and would always support one another in a conflict with nonprofessionals. Within the professional groups, physicians were most influential, although nurses at the supervisory level could often countermand the directives or priorities of interns or residents. Administration usually would concede to the top physicians, believing that what was good for medicine was good for the hospital. Within the administration the Chief Executive Officer was most influential, and power was vested in a few individuals. The Chief Executive Officer had favorites on his team and allowed these people to be privy to information and decisions denied to others. All of these cliques, favorites, and status positions were well known throughout the organization and accepted by the majority. The stated and practiced philosophy was that "we are one big family" and every family has a big daddy, favorite children, a mother, and extended relatives. The family may have its squabbles, but family always banded together against any outsiders who might threaten the family. Once accepted into the inner circle, a person's future was secure. Even though relationships may be unequal, the insiders would always be protected against outsiders. Insiders included certain secretaries and middle managers who had access to the boss and all important information. These insiders also protected the boss from "undesirables."

Socialization outside the organization was very limited. The Hospital Administrator did socialize with some of the physicians, but no other administrators were invited. Physicians and nurses likewise did not socialize except at the level of students, staff nurse and intern, or head nurse and resident. Employees did not socialize with supervisors; in fact, it was considered scandalous when such an event occurred.

Raises and promotions were based primarily on loyalty or favoritism, another fact that was well known and, in the old society, accepted. Training or development was limited to on-the-job experience, although people were assisted in obtaining additional formal education. In the old society employees were expected to care about patients, and emphasis was placed on deportment and observance of the social amenities. Discourteous behavior was not tolerated. Employees were expected to be clean and neat. Separate locker rooms were provided so that all staff including physicians and nurses could change into uniforms, which were supplied and laundered by the hospital.

Most office space, even for top executives, was very modest in size. However, the Chief Executive Officer and the Director of Nursing both had offices furnished with elegant antiques and original oil paintings. In the old society, office space was not considered a status symbol and offices were scattered all over, including the basement. Employees were expected to make appointments to see managers; there was little or no dropping-in behavior. If an employee was asked to do something, it was considered an order. Refusal of an assignment, a project, or a committee activity was not acceptable. You didn't talk back to "mom" or "dad."

Background

The nursing department, the largest single department with 1,200 full-time employees, reflected the overall organizational culture and norms. A very hierarchical, traditional organization, it also promoted very much from within. Of all the nursing administrators, only two were outsiders or nongraduates of the school associated with the medical center. Each associate director was responsible for a number of line positions (see organizational chart 1.) Staff education was centralized and included the clinicians.

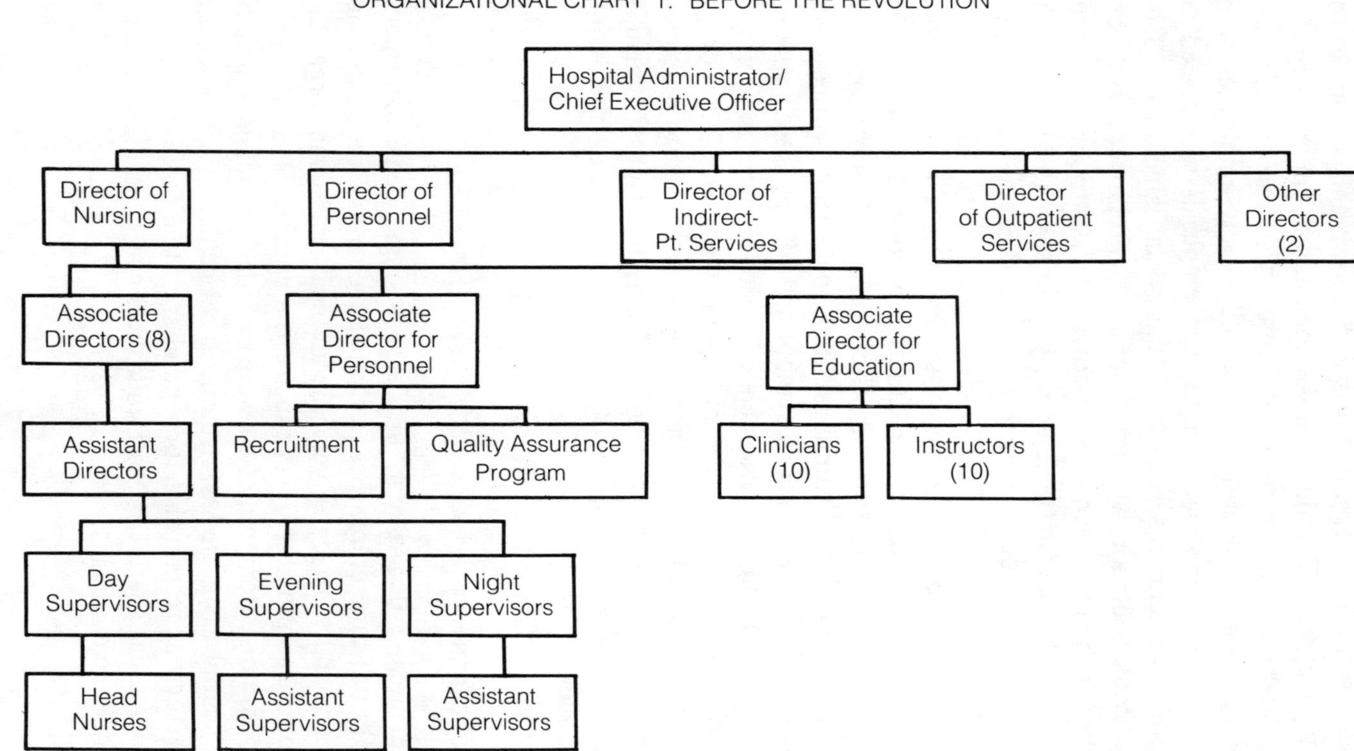
ORGANIZATIONAL CHART 1: BEFORE THE REVOLUTION
Hospital Administrator/
Chief Executive Officer
Director of
Nursing
Director of
Personnel
Director of
Indirect-
Pt. Services
Director
of Outpatient
Services
Other
Directors
(2)
Associate
Directors (8)
Associate
Director for
Personnel
Associate
Director for
Education
Assistant
Directors
Recruitment
Quality Assurance
Program
Clinicians
(10)
Instructors
(10)
Day
Supervisors
Evening
Supervisors
Night
Supervisors
Head
Nurses
Assistant
Supervisors
Assistant
Supervisors

The Director of Nursing, an insider, had been chosen from the group by her peers. She had a master's degree, as did most of the other associate directors, all of whom were over 40. Several of these associates were officers in the alumni association, a very influential group who contributed heavily to the hospital endowment fund. As previously described, many of the associates also had strong ties with influential physicians whom they had grown up with--a kind of old-boy old-girl network.

Supervisors and assistant directors were mostly bachelor's-prepared graduates from the affiliated school. Head nurses, about half of whom were graduates of the school, were mostly older, single women who were expected to be good clinicians as well as good managers. The head nurse role, however, was limited. They had no budget nor did they do staffing or hire or fire employees. These functions were part of the supervisor's responsibility. On some days, the head nurse might have to take a patient assignment, as staffing was tight.

Nursing care was organized on a team, functional, or case assignment, depending on staffing and the head nurse's preference. Almost all nurses were RNs, primarily diploma graduates. There were few LPNs, but a large group of (until recently) loyal old-time aides recruited from the neighborhood. Just before the revolution, because of the difficulties in recruiting, foreign nurses had been hired as patient care technicians or as graduate nurses on evenings and nights.

Nursing care was considered to be excellent, particularly in relation to technical skill. There was no nursing research activity and only sporadic patient teaching by the clinicians primarily. There was a heavy emphasis on continuous clinical in-service programs and conferences, but management development programs were held only periodically. There was a generous budget for outside education, but usually only top management attended conferences and conventions.

Nurses generally, although primarily viewed and described as mothers or sisters, were treated well by hospital administration. Each month the Director of Nursing and her associates had a luncheon meeting with the President and the other department directors. This meeting was both informational and problem solving. Many vested interests and hidden agendas were clarified and modified because of these meetings. The director of Nursing and the Hospital Administrator had a very positive relationship and consistently supported one another.

The Hospital Administrator decided to take an early retirement because of the many changes occurring both in the community and in the hospital business. He anticipated that there may be a need for a different organization and management style to meet the changes in client base, reimbursement sources, and employee expectations. He decided to go while he still felt good about his term as Chief Executive Officer.

The Revolution

Shortly after the Hospital Administrator's voluntary retirement, it became obvious that the hospital's financial situation was becoming desperate. Cash flow was extremely compromised because of payment lags from state government payors, changes in patient mix, and increasing costs. Unions continued to threaten inroads into both nonprofessional and professional groups. Most of the hospital systems for payroll, admissions/discharges, accounting, and laboratory data needed to be computerized, and facilities were at a point of collapse.

The Board of Trustees decided it was time to hire an aggressive administrator who would put the hospital on a sound financial basis.

Principal Players: After the Revolution

President/Chief Executive Officer (PCEO)

The new PCEO is a tough, no-nonsense administrator in his early 40s who has the reputation of being a hatchet man. He has previously been responsible for turning around several other large hospitals in financial difficulty. He has been given full authority by the Board to do whatever it will take to improve the financial situation. He is described as a "theory X type" who manages by intimidation, but gets the job done. Within a month of being hired he has forced the resignation or retirement of several directors including the Director of Nursing. He has replaced those leaving with his own people and given them all more status in title, salary, and benefits. All vice-presidents now have handsome new offices in an executive suite in a remodeled building. Rewards and security in the position are based on "bottom-line" outcomes. The PCEO's philosophy is that people are all replaceable--what counts are results.

Vice-President for Nursing

The VPN is a dynamic, attractive, enthusiastic woman in her late 30s who holds both a master's in nursing and an MBA. She has never held an administrative position in a medical center but has been a very successful Director of Nurses in a community hospital. She is sincere and ambitious. She has been charged with putting the nursing department in order and would like to make it a nationally recognized department for innovation. The VPN has made it her business to get involved in both the local community and the nursing community, something that was never a priority of previous nursing directors.

Associate Director for Education (ADE)

The ADE is a single woman in her early 40s who has come up in the ranks. She has built a strong education department that includes 10 instructors and 10 clinicians, all of whom are academically and clinically well prepared. A graduate of the nursing school affiliated with the hospital, the ADE is respected by her fellow associate directors and is very active in the alumni association.

Clinical Associate Directors (CADs)

The CADs are all middle-aged women who have earned their status through the traditional system. Although none have advanced management skills such as finance, strategic planning, or human resource development, they have managed to maintain the status quo, a previous organizational norm. None have worked anywhere else; all are financially and psychologically vested in the hospital, and few have established a life apart from it. They have dedicated their professional life to the hospital and are confused and anxious about the new regime.

The Present Situation

The VPN is determined to horizontally integrate or decentralize the nursing organization, which she believes has too many levels of administration and not enough participative management. She wants the functions of recruitment and staff development decentralized and to be implemented at the unit level by assistant patient care managers. She does not support the concept of clinicians or clinical specialists, believing they have not justified their cost. She does support and believe in a strong head nurse role and to this end has designed a new organizational chart (see organizational chart 2). Head nurses, to be called patient care managers, will report directly to the CADs and will have assistant patient care managers reporting to them. These assistants will be responsible for staff development and supervision on evenings and nights. This reorganization will eliminate the positions of assistant director, supervisor, clinician, and instructor. Patient care managers will have 24-hour accountability and be responsible for their own budget, hiring, firing, staffing, and development of their assistants.

The VPN has established many task forces and committees to write new job descriptions, performance standards, and standards for practice. She has requested that the eight associate directors submit within three months plans for consolidating the eight departments into four; that each identify their professional

ORGANIZATIONAL CHART 2: AFTER THE REVOLUTION

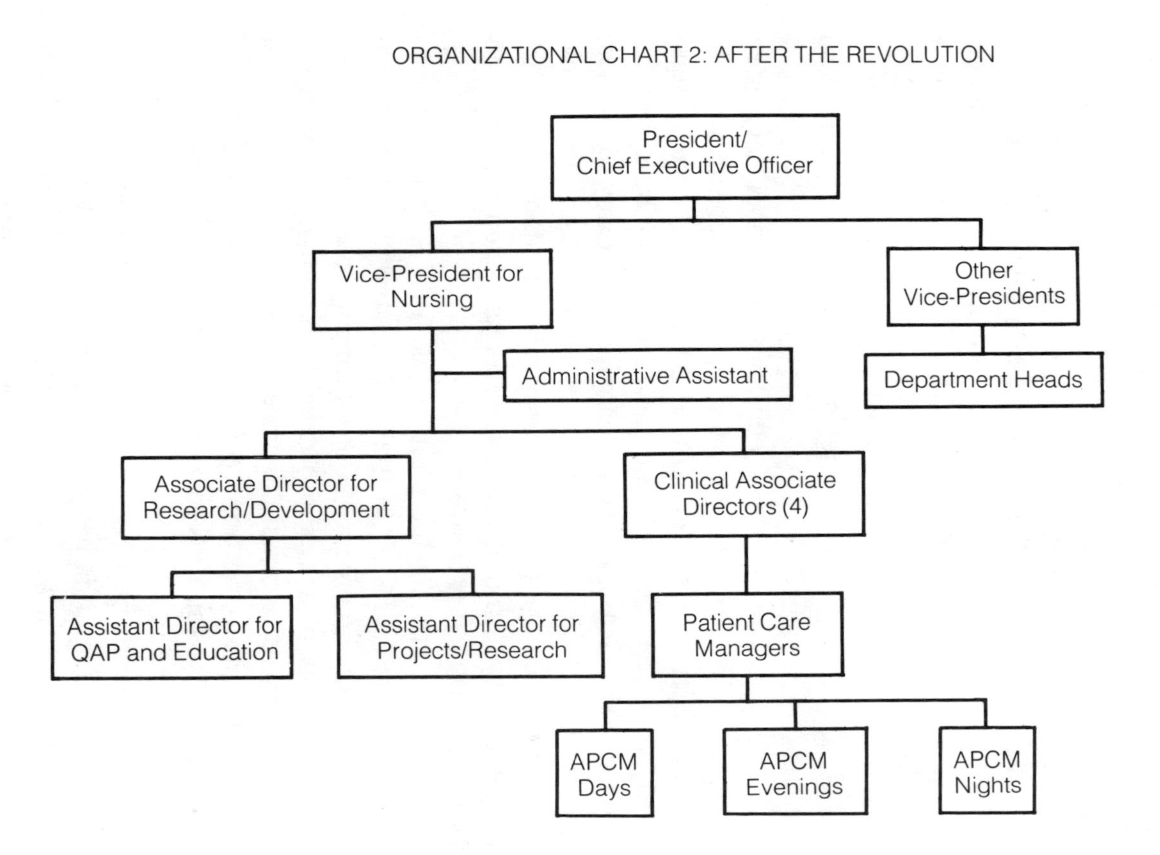

goals; and that they bid for the position they believe will be most appropriate for them in the reorganization. The VPN has promised that no one will lose salary or benefits in the reorganization; however, it is unlikely that any of the incumbents will be qualified for the new Clinical Associate Director position. One associate director has already taken early retirement.

The present ADE has been asked to submit a plan for establishing a revenue-generating continuing education function and also a program to prepare qualified head nurses for the new position of patient care manager. After the patient care manager plan has been successfully implemented, assistants will be hired, eliminating the need for supervisors on evenings and nights.

The clinicians and staff education instructors have been given the opportunity to apply for the position of either patient care manager or assistant. These 20 individuals are all relatively young and new to the organization. They have been attracted to the idea of collective bargaining as a way to promote the needs and demands of the nursing profession. In the old regime they enjoyed positions of relative freedom and self-direction. They do not perceive the reorganization to be in their best interest.

Before accepting the position, the VPN obtained a commitment from the PCEO to establish 150 new full-time staff positions for RNs in order to bring staffing up to a desirable level. The VPN has also established an open-door policy with the staff and holds a bimonthly meeting with them. No other nursing administrators are present at these meetings. The staff nurses perceive the VPN to be their champion are are very supportive of her and her ideas.

Two months have passed. There is a great deal of informal discussion of what is happening in the organization. Rumors are rampant about which nursing divisions will merge and who will remain in which position. The annual alumni meeting of the school of nursing is scheduled for next week. A special session on the reorganization has been arranged for alumni by the

ADE. Two of the CADs will be making the presentation; the VPN has not been invited.

Questions

1. Predict the success of the VPN's reorganization plan. Support your prediction with relevant facts and extrapolations.

2. What options do you think the present associate directors have for the future?

3. What are the relative advantages and disadvantages of the nursing reorganization plan?

case study 12

Complex relationships

Setting

The hospital in this case is a relatively new hospital. Groundbreaking ceremonies were held in 1954 and the hospital opened its doors in 1956. As stated in its public brochure, the hospital's mandate is " . . . to serve the community with a compelling spirit of Christian care."

The hospital is a Catholic hospital, owned by an order that operates approximately 50 health care institutions. The tenets of Catholicism and the beliefs of the order are apparent in its many documents and statements, most often expressed as their commitment to "quality Christian care."

The philosophy and beliefs espoused by the hospital fit well with the culture and beliefs of those in the community where it is located. Although located in a large industrial city, the community surrounding the hospital is best described as an Eastern European ethnic neighborhood, composed mostly of first-, second- and third-generation Polish and German Catholics. It is an old neighborhood, its homes having been built in the first part of the century. Although the neighborhood is predominantly residential, one section of the area is highly industrialized, and most residents are blue-collar workers. The neighborhood is characterized by a shared sense of common ethnicity and culture.

The hospital is a community hospital of 200 beds plus 50 bassinettes. Twenty-two years after it was built, a major renovation and expansion program began which was recently completed. Thus, it is a modern facility offering a full complement of acute care services. There are over 1,300 employees occupying 900 full-time positions. In nursing, there are 400 budgeted fulltime positions, 95% of which are filled. Most of the employees are drawn from the surrounding neighborhood, as are the patients. The patient revenue base is 42% third-party payors, 40% Medicare, 10% private-pay, and 8% Medicaid.

External Environment

Even though the community surrounding the hospital is truly a community with rather clear boundaries, it is a neighborhood within a larger city and an even larger metropolitan area. The city is divided into an east side and a west side by a large industrial valley and river; the hospital is on the west side. The bulk of health care facilities for the city are found on the east side, however, and it is estimated that 40% of the west siders go to the east side for care because they believe the quality is better there.

There are four other hospitals on the west side; three of them are community hospitals and the fourth is a growing medical center. The hospital faces additional competition: many of the east side hospitals are setting up satellite centers on the west side, and surgicenters and emergicenters are proliferating throughout the city.

The hospital has neither a bad nor a good reputation. Rather, it has a nothing reputation. Many believe that there are problems with both the medical and nursing care and practices. Furthermore, the hospital has not taken a long-range view of its external environment and competition. It has contracted for a major marketing survey, though, and the results are expected in the next six months.

Internal Environment

Both insiders, consisting of those associated with the hospital and those living within the neighborhood, as well as outsiders from the larger metropolitan area, see the hospital as an extension of the families on the west side. The strong subculture of the community pervades the internal environment, and its informal communication system is one of the best. Everyone knows everyone else and more often than not they are related. Consequently, the interaction style is appropriately informal: everyone knows and speaks to everyone else on a first-name basis, regardless of rank or position.

Fifty percent of the hospital's employees have been there since it opened. The loyal employee who cares about the hospital is the one promoted, often without regard to performance. Thus, although longevity and loyalty are intentionally rewarded, it sometimes appears that mediocrity is rewarded also.

There is a special relationship between "the hospital" (by which is generally meant hospital management, although "the hospital" is often referred to in a nebulous way) and its employees. This relationship is like a family: "the hospital" is viewed as and acts like the parent. The religious sisters, many of whom live in the convent next to the hospital and work at the hospital, are very protective of people who work at the hospital, particularly long-term employees, and care about them like family. Thus, there is a certain closeness and understanding among people, predicated on an assumption of a common ethnic belief and value system. Employees are, however, described as aggressive. Yelling, screaming, and demanding are usual behaviors. Employees are described as spoiled children who demand everything from their parents. For example, employees are provided free coffee during variable two-hour periods on each shift. This freebie costs the hospital $40,000 annually, yet employees want more. Parental management and aggressive, demanding employee behavior may appear paradoxical but are congruent with their relationship--families do bicker and argue. Because employees and the community see the hospital as "theirs," they want it to be run the way they think it ought to be. Thus, the organizational milieu is at times beneficial and at other times detrimental to the hospital's primary mission.

The organization of the hospital is centralized, and the systems of decision making and supervision are described as caste-like and authoritarian. In such a centralized system, one would expect a top-down communication pattern to predominate. The top-down pattern is a frequently used pattern, but it is second in order of frequency. The most frequent, rapid, and inaccurate communication system is the rumor mill. A bottom-up pattern is also used, but much less frequently than the other two, and is of lesser importance.

Until five years ago, the hospital enjoyed a stable management. Sisters from the order occupied key executive and management positions, including the positions of Administrator and Director of Nursing. Five years ago the hospital contracted with a national corporation for management services. This corporation brought in a President, an Executive Vice-President, a Vice-President for Nursing, and a Vice-President for Personnel Services, all of whom were employees of the national corporation approved by the hospital Board of Directors. The remaining executive and managerial positions were filled by incumbent employees.

The hospital is a centralized and traditionally structured organization. The President reports to the Board of Directors, 50% of whom are lay members drawn from the community and 50% members of the religious order. The Board reports to the religious order. Reporting to the President are seven vice-presidents: for nursing, personnel services, building services, financial services, planning and professional development, and professional services (two vice-presidents). Reporting to the vice-presidents are numerous department heads (see hospital organizational chart).

Many of the department head positions are held by nuns who have been with the hospital from its beginning. Other department head positions are held by loyal employees who have been promoted over the years. The first Director of Nursing, who had been the Director from the beginning until five years ago, is still in the organization in charge of the order's Renew program, a national program whose purpose is to examine

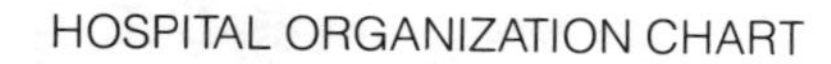
HOSPITAL ORGANIZATION CHART

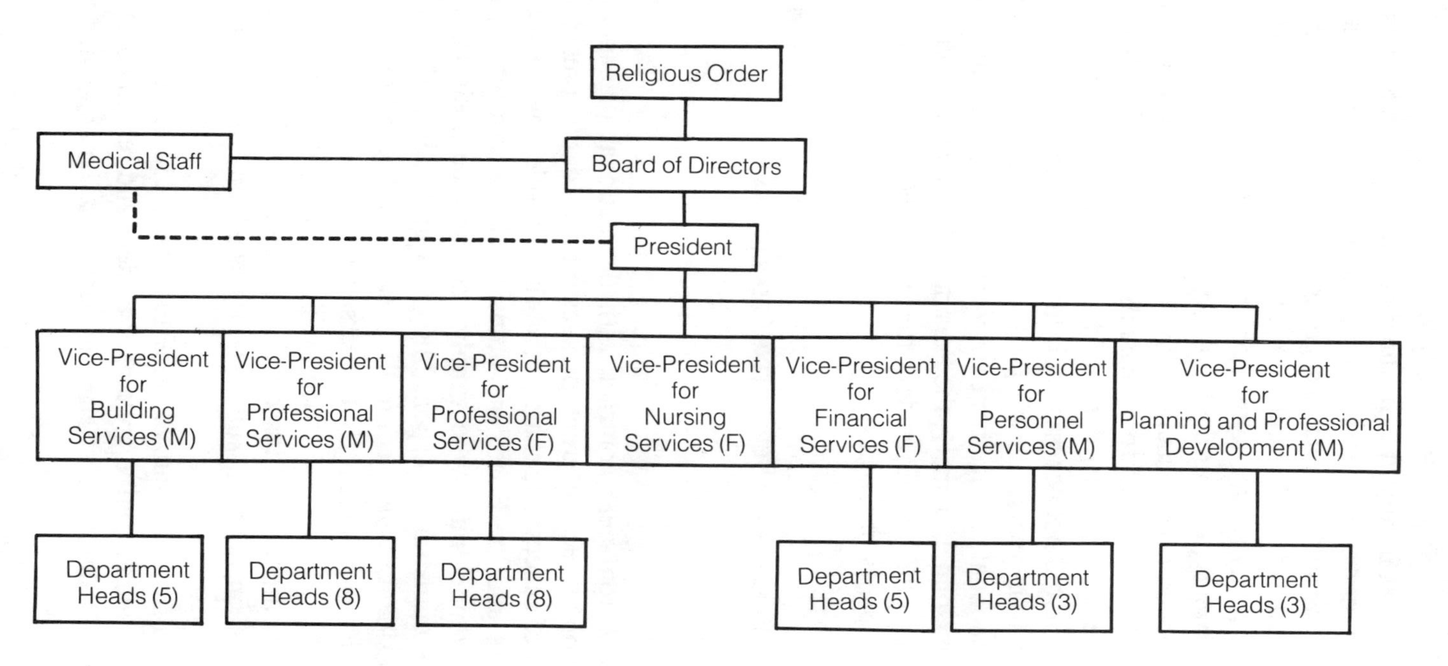
Religious Order
Medical Staff
Board of Directors
President
Vice-President for Building Services (M)
Vice-President for Professional Services (M)
Vice-President for Professional Services (F)
Vice-President for Nursing Services (F)
Vice-President for Financial Services (F)
Vice-President for Personnel Services (M)
Vice-President for Planning and Professional Development (M)
Department Heads (5)
Department Heads (8)
Department Heads (8)
Department Heads (5)
Department Heads (3)
Department Heads (3)

Catholic values in regard to health care. In line with her charge, she has set up multiple ad hoc committees and schedules meetings every week with various groups. In this way she still maintains contact with employees even though her responsibility is not directly related to the hospital's operation.

In summary, during the first 23 years of the hospital's history it enjoyed a very stable, although perhaps stagnant, management. Over the past four years its management has been far from stable, and is better described as turbulent. The change in management did not necessarily bring innovation.

After four years, the hospital will not renew its contract with the national management corporation. The national corporation's personnel, namely, the President, the Vice-President for Nursing, and the Vice-President for Personnel services, will become employees of the hospital.

Principal Players and Supporting Characters

President

During the four-year contract with the national management corporation, three different persons occupied the presidency (see line of succession chart). The first President was liked by the sisters and the Board of Directors. He was a placid, do-nothing administrator who simply occupied the position. The "real" administrative responsibility was given to the Executive Vice-President, a very controlling and secretive administrator slow in decision making. The first President lasted only two years. The Executive Vice-President was then appointed Acting President and subsequently President. The Executive Vice-President position subsequently was eliminated from the organizational chart.

The former Executive Vice-President continued his authoritative and secretive style as President and remained in the position only one year. Before his departure he appointed two

LINE OF SUCCESSION CHART

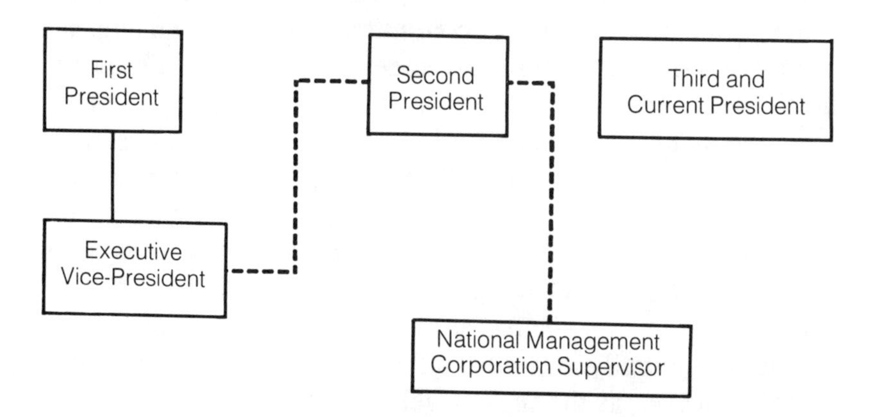

people to vice-presidential positions; these appointments were promotions from within and will be described later.

The second President subsequently became the national corporation's supervisor for the hospital, an untenable arrangement for the third President. The third President is a stark contrast to the previous presidents. On the job for only six months, he is seen as action oriented. He is very quick to make decisions and expects things to get done, an expectation foreign to employees. This President is a very candid, up-front administrator who readily shares information. He has an open-door policy toward his management team and is visible throughout the institution; he is known to "make rounds" on all shifts. Although action oriented, he is also described as impulsive, making decisions without thinking them through. He gives orders, rescinds them, and then gives new, contradictory orders.

Vice-President for Nursing (VPN)

A new VPN was appointed as part of the management contract. This person replaced the former Director of Nursing, a sister, who had been in that position since the hospital's inception. This VPN, a former clinical specialist, did not succeed. She was described as too "sophisticated" for the staff and held expectations for change that were beyond the vision of the organization at the time. Although committed to primary nursing, she could not move her staff in that direction, and made demands to the national corporation and to the nuns that could not be met.

Two years later another VPN was appointed and remains as the current VPN. Master's-prepared with a proven and credible record in nursing administration, she has been at the hospital for two years and has been able to temper her goals with the growth and development of the organization. During her two-year tenure, she has seen the first two Presidents come and go and initially viewed the third President as an improvement. However, as the stress level in the hospital increases, she now views the President as "crisis-oriented," sees his impulsiveness as destructive, and finds it difficult to predict or know for sure his policies and positions.

Other Vice-Presidents

As described earlier, two vice-presidents were appointed by the second President before his departure. The former head of radiology was appointed Vice-President of Professional Services. This appointment occurred at a time when many employees were being laid off. His qualifications for the job were a high school diploma, many years of on-the-job experience, and a recently completed BS in health administration. He is considered by some to be a "favorite son," and on completion of his degree the sisters hosted a celebration party in his honor.

The former Director of Hospital Education, also a long-time employee, was appointed Vice-President of Planning and development when the hospital education department was eliminated. The second President had groomed these two appointees in his own administrative style, controlling and secretive. Both vice-presidents are described as turf-builders and do not cooperate with others on the management team.

The Vice-President for Personnel Services came to the hospital with the national management corporation five years ago. He is committed to hospital goals but also sees its many problems.

The Vice-President for Building Services has been in his position for seven years. He is cooperative, easy to work with, and described as doing a good job.

The other Vice-President for Professional Services, a nun, is new to the position. In her early 30s, she has just completed her master's in health administration. She is viewed as someone with great potential who is being given experience on her way to higher-level positions within the health care corporation being formed by the order.

The Vice-President for Financial Services, also a nun, was at the hospital when it opened and has been there ever since. She is also the mother superior at the convent next door to the hospital. Officially, in terms of hospital business, she holds only a vice-presidential position, but informally many plans and decisions are determined by her as she represents the highest authority in the local order.

Background

The nursing environment at the hospital is influenced by the organizational milieu and community culture. Although the common culture provides a degree of cohesiveness among staff, it is also restrictive and punitive. Differences are not tolerated and there is little openness to new ideas. Indeed, differences and new ideas are usually suspected and rejected.

The latest VPN, trying to implement changes in the nursing department, is constantly plagued by a five-year, ongoing labor-management issue. The hospital used to run smoothly, or at least the employees perceive that it did so. When labor issues surfaced, "administration" began to lose credibility in the eyes of the staff, who became increasingly disgruntled with "the hospital," even though many of the changes experienced were a result of external factors. For example, as a result of President Carter's wage guidelines, the hospital altered its long-standing way of granting wage increases. This change affected the pattern of raises received by employees in this hospital and every other hospital in the community. At the same time, the nursing department, like every other nursing department in the community, had many vacancies. Staff subsequently felt overworked. This unrest and dissatisfaction resulted in repeated union-organizing campaigns by various employee groups.

Five years ago the situation came to a head. An employee attitude survey was conducted which indicated serious administrative and managerial problems. The professional nursing staff contacted several unions. When a local affiliate of one of the nonnursing unions started a strong organizing campaign among the nurses, the hospital was surprised. It had survived meager organizing efforts before and therefore did not consider unionization a real threat. In the meantime, as a result of the attitude survey, the hospital secured the services of a national management consulting firm to provide supervisory training and to help reestablish the administration's credibility. The consulting firm's members used a confronting and aggressive style. Some employees perceived the group as a union-busting firm. In the midst of this turmoil, the medical staff expressed their displeasure with various and sundry conditions and succeeded in "getting rid" of the administrator, the nun who had occupied the position since the hospital opened. All these events, plus others, led to the hospital's present contract with the management company.

Shortly after the management company took over, the professional nursing staff held an election for representation by a local affiliate of a nonnursing union. The vote was 100 against, 95 for union representation. The union filed an unfair labor practices suit and sought a bargaining order. This case has still not been decided. In four years, the national management corporation has been able neither to stabilize nor to improve the hospital environment. It is within this context that the VPN has tried to implement change.

The reputation of nursing at the hospital has not been positive. Nursing has suffered from a lack of constructive, unifying leadership over the years. Professional individuals do not stand out, nor is there a high level of professional behavior demonstrated by the staff. The new VPN, recognizing the need for fresh blood and new ideas, is trying to bring in people who demonstrate professional behavior.

When the VPN arrived two years ago, 33% of the nursing staff were RNs. At present there is a 50% RN complement. The VPN does not know the educational background of her staff, and the employee relations department will not give her this information. Although she could obtain this information by polling her staff, she does not want to raise unwarranted suspicions among her staff at this time.

Hospital staff are used to the status quo and are resistant to change. This is true not only in the nursing department, but throughout the entire hospital. The hospital has a sophisticated computer system, but because staff are task oriented, they do not see the purpose of this, only the pieces. Consequently, there is triplication of effort despite a well-designed and sophisticated system. Several of the department heads have tunnel vision and resist change. After a year of planning and discussion, a unit pharmacy system was implemented. The pharmacy set as acceptable a 15% medication error rate. Because nursing found this error rate too high and because pharmacy refused to discuss or consider any change in the standard error rate, nursing had to duplicate efforts in order to prevent such a high number of serious medication errors.

The medical staff is described as older, with an average age of over 50. The hospital has not in the past been able to attract a cadre of younger physicians. Twenty-five percent of the physicians account for 60% of patient admissions, and the majority of the medical staff hold an archaic view of nursing.

The nursing staff is, however, becoming more open to new ideas and change. For example, all nursing units have implemented the problem-oriented system of charting. Prior to implementation the VPN appointed an ad hoc committee composed of the head nurse, the unit teacher, and a staff nurse from every patient unit. This ad hoc committee planned for the problem-oriented charting system and strategized to effect a constructive change. Therefore, whenever physicians or other hospital personnel questioned or criticized the new charting system, staff supported and defended the system they felt they owned.

The nursing staff has not become fully participative and cooperative with administration, however. The VPN, in writing new philosophy, sent a draft to all the nursing staff on every unit asking for their input and comments. This was a new experience for staff, who had never before participated in the preparation of any statement or policy. No one on the staff had any comment for change. A few staff said they liked what it said. The VPN admits that the philosophy statement is rather basic and not creative or innovative, but is congruent with what the hospital and nursing staff are presently doing.

Prior to the VPN's arrival, the nursing department was very top-heavy with multiple clinical directors, shift supervisors, and head nurses. Despite the number of middle managers, the department was very centralized, with all decisions being made in the "director's office." Middle management was perceived to be punitive, restrictive, and generally poor.

The Incident

The VPN made one of her first goals decentralization of the centralized nursing organization. In the old system were five clinical directors (equivalent to supervisors), an evening and night clinical director, and a Director of Nursing Practice (DNP), who was also the day director. All of these directors reported to the VPN. In an interim and initial move, the VPN eliminated three of the clinical director positions. Two of these clinical directors were moved easily into new positions, but the third was problematic. However, since the DNP position was vacant, the VPN moved her, with reservations, into that position (see interim nursing organizational chart).

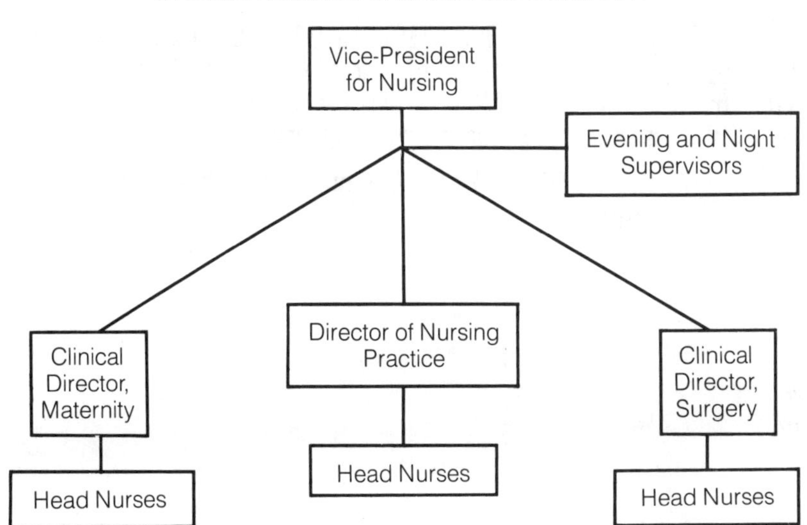

The DNP does not have a good reputation; personnel are intimidated by her and are afraid of her. She wields a great deal of informal power because of her longevity at the hospital and her being a favorite of the nuns. She is viewed as a "snoopervisor" and often punishes staff in a parent-child manner, demoting several people in a less than appropriate way. The VPN, despite her misgivings, had decided to try to work with her in this new capacity.

Six months after this appointment, it is apparent that the DNP cannot function in the position. The VPN has collected data and well documented the DNP's incompetence. Furthermore, the DNP is not supportive of the VPN and undermines her in insidious ways. To add insult to injury, the DNP earns the same salary as the VPN. The VPN has thought of moving the DNP into a vacant unit manager position, but the hospital President has closed that unit permanently. It is obvious that the DNP should be fired, but a consultant from the national management corporation has warned the VPN to use great caution as "the DNP has the nuns in her back pocket."

QUESTIONS

1. What options does the VPN have? Should she fire the DNP, move her into another position, reduce her salary, etc.? What are the benefits and risks associated with each option for the VPN personally and for the nursing organization?

2. Should the VPN discuss the situation with the influential nuns at the hospital?

case study 13

A fatal attack

SETTING

This case takes place in a 400-bed, acute care, not-for-profit community hospital located in a medium-sized city in the South. The hospital, originally built in the 1950s, has undergone considerable renovation and reconstruction. It is now a very handsome, five-story building with a large parking area and a separate doctor's office building. The hospital is very proud of having the latest in medical equipment and services. It is considered the leading hospital in the city, which has several other smaller facilities.

The hospital has an excellent reputation for providing personalized care and makes its facilities available for many community activities such as health fairs, weight and smoking programs, art contests, and social activities. The hospital auditorium, a large, attractive room, is well-used by medical and community groups.

Although there has been some increase in the number of Medicare patients over the past few years, 70% of the hospital's income is still derived from private insurance payments. Fiscal management has never been a problem and is not anticipated to be one. Although no new programs are being considered at this time, management expects that the hospital will eventually increase to about 550 beds because of community growth.

The Board of Trustees, made up of leading local citizens and executives from the many industries in the area, is very pleased with the management of the hospital and gives full support to its decisions.

External Environment

The city is an old one with a rich history. Over the past 15 years it has benefited from the influx of business from the North. Many large companies have located regional or corporate offices in the vicinity, bringing people and revenue into the area. Construction of homes and shopping centers has boomed. Most of the new businesses are nonindustrial, employing clerical, professional, and technical personnel who receive good salaries. All of these newcomers are welcomed for their business and treated cordially, but have not really been assimilated into the original culture group.

The old guard are primarily white Baptists, either old money or tradespeople. There has always been a small black minority group who work as servants or municipal workers and are described as "knowing their place." Integration is minimal, but there have been few overt racial problems. The newcomers represent a mix of religious and ethnic groups but are also primarily white. Many of the management and professional newcomers have been invited to join the country club and service organizations but are still not privy to the exclusive social organizations. There have been some disagreements between old and new in relation to increases in taxes for public schools and a new sewage system, but no serious conflicts have arisen. City government is still controlled by the old guard, who tend to be fairly conservative. Both old guard and newcomers agree that the city is a very pleasant place to live, and no one wants to make any change that would upset that feeling.

Internal Environment

Like the city itself, the hospital is considered to be a pleasant place to work. Because of its excellent financial position, salaries are competitive, equipment and supplies are always available, and employees receive a bonus every year. Many of the employees are old-guard locals who have been born and raised in the community. The atmosphere is cordial and friendly. Employees address one another as "Mrs." or "Mr." on the job, but by first name outside. Many of the employees know the patients but also address them formally while they are patients.

Rituals are important in the hospital. Employees receive a card from the executive office on their birthday, and everyone attends the annual Christmas party for employees and their families. Turkeys are given out at Thanksgiving and hams at Easter. Weddings, engagements, births, and vacation doings are reported regularly in the hospital newsletter. Even though the hospital has grown to over 2,000 employees, efforts are made to maintain the atmosphere of camaraderie. No employees are unionized, and there has been no union activity in the hospital.

Personnel are rewarded for their support of this atmosphere and for maintaining the reputation of the hospital as a warm, caring agency. The hospital is very proud of being modern and up-to-date and promotes individuals who are also up-to-date, but within the style of the organization. Every effort is made to promote from within, but the organization will go outside for the right person.

Reflecting the ethnic mix in the community, there are few nonwhite employees. Individuals are trained on the job primarily. There is a nursing in-service department and a large fund for sending managers and some staff to continuing education meetings. All levels of employees are encouraged to go to the annual regional hospital association convention, and buses are provided to transport people to this meeting. The hospital supports a school for LPNs, established 25 years ago. The school has a good reputation and graduates approximately 30 nurses per year, all of whom usually pass state board examinations on their first attempt. Many of these graduates work in the hospital.

The organization is a traditional, centralized structure. Management style is also traditional with communication flowing from the top down. There is opportunity, however, for employees to communicate concerns and suggestions, and most people describe the management as fair and reasonable. There are the usual kinds of rules and policies, but no one gets too strict about enforcing them unless there is a real problem. Considering the size of the organization, there are relatively few serious organizational problems. The biggest issue in the past year was whether or not to substitute vending machines for cafeteria hours at certain times of the day.

Principal Players and Supporting Characters

Chief Executive Officer (CEO)

The CEO is a male in his early 60s who has been with the hospital for 40 years. He has come up from the ranks and has seen the hospital grow from 200 beds to its present size. Although he has no formal education beyond a bachelor's degree, he has kept up-to-date on theories and practices of hospital administration. The CEO is described as a good old boy and is well liked. As part of the local old guard he knows everyone who is anyone in the community and has connections everywhere. His management style is loose, letting his managers run their departments without interference unless there is a problem. He uses compromise and negotiation frequently to resolve differences and does not play favorites. He has let it be known that he will retire in two years and is grooming his Associate Administrator for the position, but would also support selection of someone else from the outside if the Board thought it better.

Associate Administrator (AA)

The AA, in his late 30s, is also a local old-guard male. He has an MBA and is described as a "comer." Very ambitious, he takes his responsibilities and himself very seriously. He spent two years in a medical center as an assistant administrator before coming back home four years ago to this hospital. He feels that the organization could do with a tighter structure and control. He respects the CEO but feels he lets people take advantage of him. He was also very upset that, two years ago, the CEO acceded to the new Director of Nursing's request that her position report directly to the CEO instead of to the AA as it had in the past.

The AA is married to a local old-guard member who is head of the hospital LPN program.

Director of Nursing (DON)

The DON is a newcomer to the city. She is a very attractive widow in her late 30s who was recruited through a search firm to replace the retiring DON. The DON, master's-prepared, is a northerner and a member of a minority religious group. She wears high-fashion clothes to work--a first for nursing administration--and is very vivacious and quick. She is popular with her staff and most of her supervisors, who believe it was time for a change to someone who would promote nurses and nursing in the hospital.

As indicated, the DON took the job only when it was agreed that she would report directly to the CEO, not to the AA. She believed this to be important both to her personally and for the nursing department.

The DON has been in the position now for two years and has instituted change slowly. She has established herself in the professional nursing groups and has become acquainted with the directors of nursing in the other hospitals in the city. She has established a nursing practice council in the hospital and uses this as a forum for nursing practice issues and concerns. Although some people describe her as "pushy," most people think she had done good things for nursing.

One year ago she married the Director of Medical Staff.

Director of Medical Staff (DMS)

The DMS is a handsome, old-guard internist in his late 50s who was widowed about three years ago. Considered an excellent physician, he admits about 40% of the hospital's patients. He is beloved by everyone as a wonderful person, and is respected by his fellow physicians, who support his decisions even when they don't agree with him. He and the CEO are social friends as well as hospital colleagues and get along very well. The DMS is President of the Medical Board and a voting member of the Board of Trustees.

Since marrying the DON, he indulges her in everything she wants both in the hospital and outside. This is resented by many, who don't overtly resist because of their affection and respect for the DMS. There is considerable rumbling, however, in certain circles about how she is taking advantage of him.

Chief of Surgery (CS)

The CS is a 40-year-old male who was recruited five years ago from the outside because of his brilliant surgical record in cardiovascular surgery. He has started an open heart program that has been very successful medically and financially. The CS is also President-elect of the medical board, to succeed the DMS next year. The CS is described as somewhat arrogant and high-handed and has very old-fashioned ideas about nurses' place in the hierarchy. He has formed an alliance with the AA, who promotes and facilitates his programs in the hospital and has sponsored his membership in several important community groups. The CS's wife and the AA's wife have also become good friends.

Director of the LPN Program (DLPN)

The DLPN is an attractive woman in her early 30s who is a member of the old-guard society. She received a baccalaureate degree in teaching and decided on a career when she and the AA were unable to produce a family. The fact that she is not a nurse has caused some problems with the state board of nursing, but so far the school has been approved in spite of this. Her Assistant Director is a master's-prepared nurse. Many of the DLPN's friends are daughters of physicians or of members of the Board of Trustees. The DLPN treats the DON with courtesy but does not like her northern ways.

Background

When the DON took over two years ago, the nursing department was a traditional, functional service that provided good bedside care, although somewhat technical. Although all units are well staffed, the mix of nursing personnel was about 50% RNs, 40% LPNs, and 10% auxiliary. The DON has wanted to change this to a higher proportion of RNs and fewer LPNs. There is an associate degree program in the area, and quite a few of the new-guard wives moving into the community are RNs interested in part- or full-time employment. The DON has moved slowly on this issue so far. She first had the nursing offices moved to the administrative suite and furnished them with handsome furniture, paintings, and plants. She also reorganized the department by making the nursing titles consistent with other department managers and giving them authority to go with their responsibility. She has not replaced anyone but has shifted people around to make better use of their skills. She has hired several new staff development people and wants to implement an aggressive training and development function.

Her only clinical problems have been with the CS, with whom she has had several run-ins about the proper function and practice of nurses. The CS wants to dictate what nurses can and cannot do in the intensive care surgical unit. So far the DON has won most of the battles, but she knows there will be ongoing problems because there are plans to expand the open heart and vascular surgery programs.

Since marrying the DMS, the DON has requested and gotten voting membership on several medical board committees. This is resented by many physicians, who don't believe a nurse should vote, but they have gone along because of the DMS. Several wives of these same physicians also resent the DON because of their previous friendship with the DMS's first wife, a local old-guard member. These wives don't like the DON being part of their social world, but again they go along because of the DMS.

The Incident

The DON is ready now to make her move in relation to nursing staff mix. She has developed a plan for reducing the percentage of LPNs through attrition. She has a commitment from the director of the associate degree program to use the hospital for clinical practice and in return give free tuition for three courses to LPNs from the hospital. The associate degree program director has also promised to provide a challenge exam, awarding college credits to LPNs who pass the exam. The positions released through attrition and people attending the associate degree program would then be filled by RNs and aides, changing the mix to 70% RNs, 10% LPNs, and 20% auxiliary. The projected financial cost of this mix, plus a generous tuition plan for LPNs electing to upgrade, is no greater than the current salary costs. The plan also includes closing the LPN program and reallocating the classrooms and teaching resources to staff development and patient education use, a favorite project of the CEO.

The CEO has promised to support the proposal and is presenting it to the Board of Trustees. The nursing practice council is in favor of the proposal as long as no one is fired. The LPNs have mixed feelings about the proposal, but many of the younger ones are positive about the opportunity to upgrade their position at the hospital's expense.

The DMS has promised to use his influence with the Board of Trustees to get approval of the proposed plan. Voting on the plan takes place next week. All seems to be working in the DON's favor.

Two days before the scheduled Board meeting, the DMS suffers a massive myocardial infarction and, despite heroic medical efforts, dies in the emergency room.

Questions

1. What are the chances for the DON's proposed plan being approved?
2. Forecast the future of the DON in the hospital.

case study 14

The plight of the clinical specialist

SETTING

The setting for this case is a county institution complex, which includes a 200-bed acute care facility, a 600-bed long-term care facility, a 100-bed geropsychiatric facility, a 200-bed inpatient psychiatric service, and outpatient or ambulatory care facilities. Construction for 200 additional long-term beds and a massive mental health center is under way. It is an old institution located on a large campus of spacious lawns and trees. Its many buildings speak to its many generations: they reflect the changing stages of the institution's history, some standing as they were originally built, some remodeled, and some newer, more modern additions.

The facility is located in a large suburban area, surrounded by other county facilities, a dense residential area, and a sprawling commercial shopping area. The county is a wealthy one, serving as a bedroom community for a large metropolitan city. Because the county is on the border between two states, its chief identity is with the other state. In terms of the state as a whole, the county is an island--a rich county that the state has to tolerate. The county's power comes from its tax base.

The institution dates from the turn of the century, when it was a hospital for communicable disease and tuberculosis, an "old people's home," and an almshouse. Over time, its acute care services grew, and it became known as a welfare hospital and long-term care facility. Its psychiatric division grew because the county was critical of the state facility. Consequently, it is an institution with roots in "welfare cases" and socially unacceptable diseases--tuberculosis, mental illness, and aging.

When the institution began, it was located "out in the country" on a large plot of land out of the public eye. However, after World War II, the agency grounds became the center of county activity, being quickly surrounded by five elegant shopping centers all within a one-half-mile radius of the grounds. It also became a very populated residential area. About 20 years ago the county decided to concentrate more of its services on the grounds. Across the road from the institution are such facilities and services as day care, vocational education, youth housing, the county museum, and garages for county vehicles.

The image of the institution continues as one with negative connotations: a county facility. Its 200 acute beds are underutilized, operating at about 58% capacity with a considerable number of the acute care beds occupied by longer-stay patients with disposition problems. Other acute care beds serve the episodic care needs of the aged, who are transferred internally from the long-term care division. Still other acute care beds serve the very poor with alcohol, addiction, and other chronic problems with acute exacerbations. The acute care division offers low-level technology and is often used as a dumping ground for "undesirable" patients.

Because of all these factors, the acute care division is in jeopardy. Until now the philosophy of the administration has been that in spite of low technology and lack of sophistication, care has been "decent." Therefore, the administration has attempted to modify the public's negative perception. However, some believe that the division should become a center for the acute care of the aged and chronically ill, more attuned to the population that the facility attracts.

External Environment

Within a stone's throw of the county grounds are four large hospitals: a medical center, a religious-sponsored hospital, and two nonprofit community hospitals. They all offer high-tech acute care and cater to community-based physicians. All place a heavy emphasis on positive ambience--they are nice, clean, attractive hospitals. "Profit-making patients" are attracted to these hospitals. There are also several other nursing homes in the area. Most maintain a minimal number of Medicaid beds, some even refuse Medicaid patients, and some are elitist and cater solely to private-pay patients.

Every patient at the county institution has an attending physician--there are few institutionally-based physicians. The attendings are primarily semiretired physicians or foreign physicians who are attempting to establish a practice. The "premier" physicians are found in the area's competing hospitals. Transfers from the long-term care division to the acute care division are high, probably a function of the proximity of the facilities and the difference in per diem and physician reimbursement rates.

Internal Environment

Like other municipal institutions, the hospital is accountable to a Board of Freeholders, publicly elected officials who govern not only the hospital and related health facilities but other county facilities and services (see management hierarchy chart). Reporting to the Board of Freeholders and directly responsible for hospital affairs is a Board of Managers. Over the years, the Board of Managers has been able to attract good, capable management people, many of whom were sensitive to nursing and health issues. Also over the years there has been constant debate as to who controls the institution, the elected Board of Freeholders or the appointed Board of Managers. The hospital has been a "politically controlled institution" because of the persistent arguing between the Freeholders and the Managers

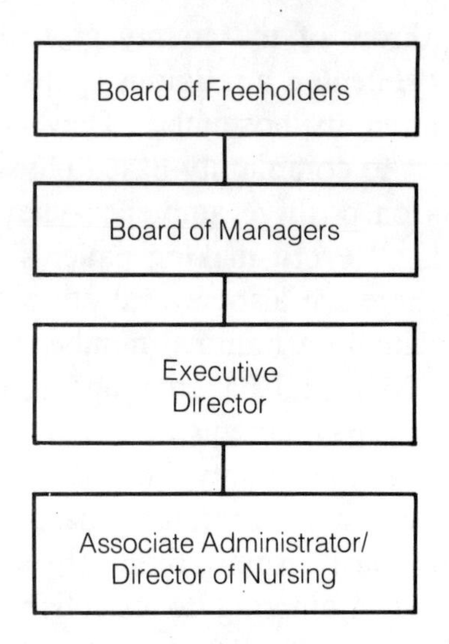

regarding authority and control and frequent interference by the Board of Freeholders, even in internal affairs.

Because the facility is a political institution, many employees are there because of political favors. A good proportion are long-service employees, including both nonprofessionals as well as professionals. The organizational structure is bureaucratic and centralized. Decision making emanates from the top down.

The educational preparation of many of the RNs is outdated, and staff development has not been a priority. The institution relies heavily on nonprofessionals; professionals and nonprofessionals are frequently used interchangeably. RNs are described as "afraid to use their muscles."

Principal Players and Supporting Characters

Executive Director

The Executive Director has been with the institution for about 10 years. In his mid-50s, he is seasoned by many wins and losses in his career. He is, of course and by necessity, very political. He wants to do well by the institution but does not want to rock the boat too much and put his job in jeopardy. He is generally supportive of nursing, but would not support nursing at the expense of antagonizing the medical staff. He was at one time quite influential with the Board of Managers, but his power and influence with this group has been eroding.

Associate Administrator/Director of Nursing (DON)

Succeeding a DON of 25 years tenure, the present DON is 40 years old and has come up through the ranks at the institution. She had been a head nurse and has held a staff development position. She holds a master's in nursing administration and is viewed as rather progressive. She is known to have good interpersonal relationships, both with administration and with the rank and file. She is also very active in outside professional activities and the state nurses' association.

Associate Director of Nursing: Administrative Affairs (ADN/AA)

The ADN/AA has been with the institution for many years and is nearing retirement age. She is rather traditional in her beliefs and background. Diploma-prepared, the ADN/AA likes things the way they were in the "good old days." Despite her traditionalism, she has been supportive of the new DON and her ideas and new programs.

Background

Shortly after taking her position, the new DON established a five-to-seven-year plan for the department of nursing which included two long-range objectives. The first objective was to incorporate clinical specialists into the organization since there were none on staff; the second was to decentralize the nursing organization.

The new DON immediately began to hire clinical specialists, whom she initially placed in a staff relationship. Her intention was to gradually, over the course of five years, move the clinical specialists into supervisory line positions. She would accomplish this by replacement of other supervisors through the normal course of attrition. The clinical specialists when hired understood that his was her intent.

The DON's plan for decentralization was not as well defined in the beginning since she did not intend to implement a decentralization model for seven years. Therefore, she modified the existing structure to the one illustrated in the nursing organization chart. It was her intent to eventually eliminate the supervisory line.

The Assistant Director/Long Term Care (ADN/LTC) was very supportive of the DON's plan and goals. Within five years of the new DON's arrival, the ADN/LTC had attracted five well-qualified clinical specialists. These clinical specialists had contributed a great deal to the quality of care provided in the long-term facility and to the education and development of staff. They had also helped develop several new clinical programs for long-term care patients. However, because the persons occupying the supervisory positions were not vacating their positions as anticipated, thereby making way for the clinical specialists to move into line positions, the ADN/LTC attempted another strategy. She decided to team up supervisors and clinical specialists; in essence, she gave joint line responsibility to a supervisor/clinical specialist team. It was her hope that the clinical specialists would help the supervisors develop more clinical skills, and at the same time the supervisors would help the clinical specialists develop management skills.

This system worked for only a short period of time. Both the clinical specialists and the supervisors found it difficult to divide responsibilities for the same areas of concern. Therefore, four of the clinical specialists resumed staff positions while one of them moved into a vacated supervisory posi-

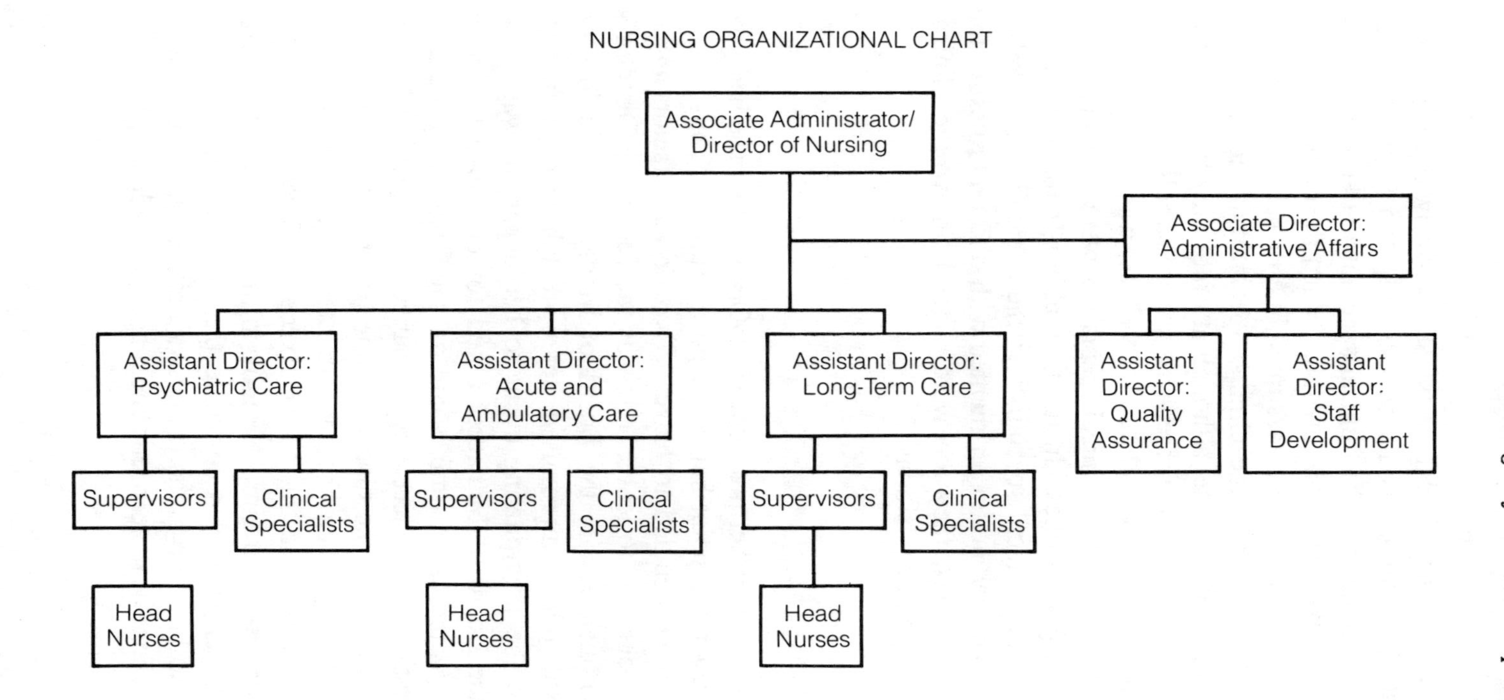
NURSING ORGANIZATIONAL CHART
Associate Administrator/
Director of Nursing
Associate Director:
Administrative Affairs
Assistant Director:
Psychiatric Care
Assistant Director:
Acute and
Ambulatory Care
Assistant Director:
Long-Term Care
Assistant
Director:
Quality
Assurance
Assistant
Director:
Staff
Development
Supervisors
Clinical
Specialists
Supervisors
Clinical
Specialists
Supervisors
Clinical
Specialists
Head
Nurses
Head
Nurses
Head
Nurses

tion. However, the clinical specialists, who now once again occupied staff positions, would occasionally and temporarily assume a line position. The clinical specialists, like the supervisors, worked weekends on rotation. When the clinical specialists worked weekends, they assumed line or house supervisory responsibilities. Thus, the clinical specialists functioned in a staff role most of the time, although at times they functioned in a line role. Because the shared-line supervisor/clinical specialist team notion did not work, the ADN/LTC was anxious to devise another plan. The clinical specialists were also anxious to have line responsibilities. In addition, although the assistant directors and the clinical specialists in the acute care and ambulatory services had not experimented with different roles for the clinical specialists, they too were eager to move the clinical specialists into line positions.

The Incident

After five years in her position, the DON felt that she had gotten to a desirable point but could go no further. Thus, out of frustration she decided to leave. Two primary factors influenced her decision to leave: one was the Executive Director's loss of influence with the Board of Managers. His loss of power, she felt, compromised her own sphere of influence. However, the precipitating event to her departure was more overt: the Board of Managers asked for cuts in the nursing budget. At the same time, some on the Board of Managers were questioning the necessity for supervisors. The DON had wanted to eliminate the supervisor line (most of whom were old guard), but only when she had attracted enough clinical specialists. Because she trusted the Executive Director, she conveyed these plans to him. He took to the idea like a dog to a bone and wanted her to eliminate the line immediately. She preferred to be more humane and wait and let the supervisors, many of whom were near retirement age, go gradually.

Even though it was an administrative issue and not a policy issue, and against the DON's advice, the Executive Director took his plan to eliminate supervisors immediately to the Board of Managers. He presented the idea in such a way that it appeared the only logical thing to do in order to cut costs. Because the DON's authority was compromised not only by this action but also by the Executive Director's decreasing influence, she left.

The ADN/AA with the institution for over 20 years, was appointed Acting Director. Loyal to the institution and nearing retirement, she willingly assumed the acting position. She was hopeful that a new director would be found before the date of her anticipated retirement, but if not, she would do what needed to be done. Her objective for her short tenure as Acting Director was to keep the place at peace and to keep the former DON's programs going.

Because the former DON had delegated responsibility, authority, and control to her assistant directors, the nursing department ran smoothly in her absence. She had created a number of clinical specialist positions, all filled with competent nurses who were satisfied with their jobs, except that many of them were anxious to move into line positions. Even so, the DON's departure had some effects on the nursing department. The assistant directors in particular felt the loss of her support. Nursing staff throughout the institution, who felt that the DON had represented them and nursing like no one else had before, felt bereft. Thus, although the department ran smoothly, the nursing staff and its leadership felt abandoned, without a source of support, representation, and direction. To complicate matters, nursing staff were not initially aware of the Board of Managers' decision to eliminate supervisory positions.

Shortly after the DON left, the Executive Director accelerated her decentralization plan. He had several arguments in favor of decentralization. First, in principle he felt that decentralized structure was a more effective one for a nursing department than any other. Second, he was aware of the trend in nursing to decentralize and felt that this was a good way to attract qualified and competent nurses. Third, he recognized that head nurses were being paid a very high salary and believed that head nurse responsibilities should reflect this salary. Therefore, by fiat the Executive Director eliminated all supervisory positions within the nursing department. In keeping with civil service policies, he rechanneled all the current supervisors into other positions. Some of them assumed head nurse positions while a few, who were close to retirement, resigned or retired early.

As a result of the Executive Director's action, the responsibilities and activities of the supervisors were bumped up to the assistant directors and down to the head nurses. Neither group was prepared for the realignment of responsibilities, and both felt overworked and unqualified for the jobs they had to take on.

The clinical specialists were also upset with the decision. They had been hired with the expectation that they would assume line positions; now those positions had been eliminated. They asked what their roles would be: would they be limited to staff positions or was there some other line position for them? The nursing leadership, namely, the Acting Director and the assistant directors, were not able to speak to the clinical specialists' questions and concerns. Nor were they able to develop any plans for implementing a decentralized structure or deal with the changes in their own jobs. Consequently, the clinical specialists filed a class action grievance.

Questions

Regarding the grievance:

1. As the Acting Director, how would you respond to the grievance?
2. Do the clinical specialists have a legitimate basis for their grievance?

Regarding the Executive Director's decision:

1. Should the Executive Director have waited until a new Director of Nursing had been hired before implementing his decision to eliminate the supervisory position?

2. What role(s) and position(s) could you define for the clinical specialists?

3. What plans would you make for easing the transition from a centralized structure to a decentralized one?

case study 15

Lost in a dream

SETTING

Mills Center, a residential retirement center, was founded before the turn of the century. Today it could be loosely referred to as a life care center. However, since it originated before the life care concept was articulated, Mills Center refers to itself as a residential retirement home.

The center is located near the heart of a large city and is within close proximity to two medical centers. The original structure remains today, surrounded of course by three-quarters of a century's worth of growth: two hotels, an apartment complex, two churches, numerous large homes now converted to apartments and offices, a pizza parlor, a drugstore, a dry cleaning establishment, and a bar. The facility sits on a major and congested thoroughfare leading to the center of the city. Despite its location and age, it is relatively unknown to either the professional or the lay community in its immediate environment.

The center was endowed by a wealthy citizen of the area to provide a haven for those elderly persons who, by whatever circumstances of fate, could no longer provide for their own shelter and care. Residents of the home pay a monthly fee based on their ability to pay, but such revenues do not cover all operating costs; endowment income is being used to cover deficit spending.

Responsibility for "the home" rests with a Board of Directors. The Board is composed primarily of wealthy women from the suburbs who volunteer their time. Most of these women, now elderly themselves, have averaged about 30 years on the Board. The Chairman of the Board has occupied her position for 20 years. Over the past two years two new members have been added to the Board, a woman from a nearby university and the first male. It is safe to conclude, however, that these new Board members do not wield much influence.

External Environment

The home exists almost in isolation from its external environment. It is unnoticed by the outside world. It has no real competition. Most new life care communities appeal to those who can afford to pay, and the home has a different mission. The complexity of the changing health care environment has affected the home in two major ways in recent years: it has not been able to recruit qualified professionals, and it has not been getting reimbursement for the health services it provides residents. The latter was a stimulus for a major expansion program, which is described below.

Internal Environment

The home had not undergone any major change until two years ago. Through the years, the facility has of course been refurbished, but physical changes have not been significant. The home is a two-story structure with a capacity for 90 residents. Residents have single rooms and share communal bathrooms. There is a central dining room and there are several "living room" areas. Personnel offices are also located within the home.

An Administrator is responsible for the day-to-day management of the facility. Working for the Administrator are a social worker/recreation therapist, several people in the business office, a Director of Nursing, and a personal caregiver. Other personnel are involved in housekeeping, maintenance, and food service. Since the number of personnel is minimal, the structure of the organization is neither centralized nor decentralized but may be either at any given time. The Administrator is usually the top official, but after that the lines get fuzzy. Minor issues often go directly to the Administrator, and major issues often go to several people at once. It is not unusual to find the Board Chairperson or some other Board member at the home giving directions on how to do what for a given matter.

All personnel refer to each other on a first-name basis. Despite the informality, there are lines of class and ethnicity. The Administrator, the Director of Nursing, and the social worker are all white; the other personnel are black. All Board members are addressed formally as "Miss" or "Mrs." The line of class between the Board and personnel, even administrative personnel, is clearly emphasized by Board members.

The personal caregiver is responsible for assisting residents who need help with their personal care. She came to the home with her warmth and sensitivity for older persons her only credentials and was trained on the job. The Director of Nursing is responsible for supervising the care provided by the personal caregiver, following up on residents' health problems and referring patients to and coordinating care with the physician who works with the home. When necessary, residents are referred to a nearby hospital, but they are not transferred to other nursing homes. If residents need intermediate, skilled, or terminal nursing care, this care is provided for them at the home.

In the past, the home provided primarily custodial care. It was never Medicare certified, but was Medicaid certified. In recent years, however, Mills Center was denied Medicaid recertification because it did not have the capacity to provide skilled and intermediate care. More and more of its residents needed this care, but the home could not receive reimbursement because it was not certified. This situation prompted the Board of Directors to embark upon a major change in mission and expansion.

The Board conducted a fund-raising campaign and built a new 120-bed skilled and intermediate care facility adjacent to the home. The new facility would be used to care for residents of the home; they would also admit patients to the facility from "outside." This expansion represented a significant change for the home, its first major change since its beginning. Neither the Board nor the management of the home was prepared for the increased scope and complexity that accompanied this expansion.

PRINCIPAL PLAYERS AND SUPPORTING CHARACTERS

Chairperson of the Board

The Chairperson of the Board is a wealthy and long-standing citizen of a nearby prestigious suburb. She is 70 years old and has been involved with the home for over 40 years. In fact, the home is her passion, and she devotes endless hours on its behalf. Her fondest memories of the home date back to the 1940s when she first got involved with the home. Things were less complex then. She couldn't really understand why the home was denied reimbursement, but, in her mind, if the new facility was necessary, she would be committed to it. Also, in her mind, running the home was not much different from running her own household--a little bigger perhaps, but not much different. To her, managing the new facility was just an extension of the same thing.

The Chairperson commanded a lot of power. Her word was final. She often made policy decisions without consulting the full Board, and no one on the Board questioned her authority to do so. The Secretary of the Board, another long-standing member, often disagreed with the Chairperson. She would discuss her differing opinions privately and informally with some staff but never disagreed with or confronted the Chairperson publicly. It is safe to say that the Chairperson "ran the show."

Administrator

The Administrator of the facility, a clergyman, is 45 years old and has been with the home for 12 years. Prior to his coming, the Board had searched long and hard for an administrator. Over the years, the Administrator learned that he served at the whim and pleasure of the Board. He was careful not to overstep his prerogatives and maintained a relationship of propriety with Board members. The Administrator was sincerely interested in the welfare of the residents--his heart was in the right place--but he had no training in the health care field nor in management. When the home was small, he and the other staff managed to muddle through. With the new expansion, however, the Administrator found himself often overwhelmed.

Harboring a secret love for architecture and construction, the Administrator found a safe niche in supervising and overseeing the construction of the new facility. His involvement in the "new building" became so time-consuming that he no longer concerned himself with the day-to-day operations of the home and with program and financial planning for when the new facility would open.

Attending Physician

A physician from a nearby university acted as the home's attending physician, but in fact came to the home as little as possible. No one was quite sure what else he did. The Board thought of him as "the doctor." In fact, he was the only other person associated with the home whom the Board considered to be of equal status as themselves. The Board viewed him with special favor because he had somehow singlehandedly raised a large sum of money for the new expansion effort.

Director of Nursing

The Director of Nursing is a 35-year-old diploma graduate who has been at the home for three years. Prior to her coming, there had been several years of rapid turnover in the position followed by a hiatus of time when the position was unfilled. The Administrator searched high and low and considered himself most fortunate to have found anyone. Part of the problem was the Board, who wanted to have the director of nursing "live in" as directors had done in years past. The new Director of Nursing made a good adjustment to the home and to working with the Attending Physician. Some would say that she did the doctor's work for him. She would "write up" his charts and change medications so that he could breeze in and merely sign charts. However, the Director of Nursing did bring some order to the chaos surrounding health services, and when new patient care assistants had to be hired for the new facility, she did the hiring and training. She also recruited a nurse friend to staff the new facility.

THE INCIDENT

Shortly after the opening of the new facility, a nearby school of nursing approached the home in regard to using the facility for a geriatric clinical experience site for its students. In return, the school agreed to provide the time of one of its faculty to help the home develop its health care services. (The home had to quickly prepare for a Medicaid certification site visit.)

The Board and the Administrator agreed to this arrangement, and the nurse faculty member began working at the home. The nurse faculty member, master's-prepared, was an extremely competent clinician and had had several experiences working with institutions like this one. The Director of Nursing did not like the new arrangement, however. She was threatened by the new nurse and antagonism developed almost immediately.

Over several months, the nurse faculty member went to the Administrator with citations and evidence of the Attending Physician's incompetence and oversight and the Director of Nursing's cover-up. The Administrator was reluctant to do anything about the situation. He was aware of the Attending

Physician's favored status with the Board and knew that if push came to shove, he, not the doctor, would be the one to go. Sometimes the Administrator would refer the matter back to the Director of Nursing, which resulted in more cover-up and a stronger coalition between them.

The nurse faculty member was frustrated but not impatient. She described care at the home as "nursing the charts, not nursing the patients." In a three-day rampage, the Director of Nursing and her nurse friend nursed the charts, and the home was granted temporary certification by Medicaid. According to the nurse faculty member, however, things got worse instead of better. Nursing care was bad and medical care was even worse--it was unsafe and incompetent.

The nurse faculty member spent many hours discussing the situation with the Administrator, who eventually became sympathetic to her viewpoint. The Board Secretary was also involved in a couple of their discussions and agreed to help. The nurse faculty member and the Administrator also went so far as to plan their strategy as to how to deal with the Board and the Attending Physician. Yet, after several months and after continual discussions and promises from the Administrator, the nurse faculty member has seen no action. She is now at the end of her patience and ready either for drastic action or to give up.

Questions

1. What factors contribute to the Administrator's inaction?

2. Should the nurse faculty member work through the Director of Nursing?

3. On the next Medicaid certification site visit, should the nurse faculty member blow the Attending Physician's cover?

4. Should the nurse faculty member go directly to the Board of Directors and/or the Chairperson?

PART III

Analysis of Selected Cases

How the Cases Were Developed

The questions at the end of this section were used by the authors in eliciting information for the case studies and were developed to provide a consistent pattern for development of the cases. This purposeful control results in an obvious bias in all of the cases, reflecting the authors' values and beliefs about organizational culture, power, and relationships among internal and external settings. Certainly, there may have been significant information in the actual situations not included in the stories as presented here. All of us, listeners and narrators, have selective perception and memory of what is being said or of what is going on. Therefore, even the responses we received to the questions may have been more or less reliable. Also, in some of the cases, considerable time elapsed between the actual episode and the retelling of the story. Thus, although these cases reflect reality they are also, to a greater or lesser extent, a distortion of reality. Any explanation or understanding of the cases or the events will be subject to both the reader's and the authors' perceptions.

Five representative cases have been analyzed by the authors as examples of how the events of the stories might be interpreted or explained. Each analysis follows the same format, which is based on selected variables and biases related to power, politics, and organizational culture. The variables identified as important were cultural norms, individual and group values, and sacred cows; relationships and power needs; hidden agendas and vested interests; and timing and external environmental factors.

Readers will notice that the majority of the cases describe unsuccessful attempts to deal with power, politics, or culture in the various organizations. This skewing is not representative of the world of nursing administration at large, where many nurse executives manage their worlds very successfully. Rather, the authors believe these cases to be relevant examples of what can go wrong--and they also make good stories.

If these cases are to be used for educational purposes, the authors suggest that instructors develop a similar format for analysis of each of the remaining cases. An alternative approach would be the development of a model answer format including significant variables/factors, differentiation of variables that could have been changed or manipulated from those that are fixed or immutable, and optional strategies to achieve a different, more desirable outcome.

Another approach for analysis could involve the use of an entirely different conceptual view of organizational dynamics. Since the cases are based on actual complex situations, multiple interpretations of the events and their sequelae are possible.

Lastly, the cases may be read simply for a better understanding or validation of the risks, challenges, and complexities involved in nursing service administration.

Questions Used to Elicit the Case Studies

Setting

- ***Size.*** Is the agency a large one, a small one, medium-sized? What is the number of beds? Of personnel?

- ***Location.*** Is the agency located in an urban, suburban, or rural setting? In what part of the country is it located?

- ***Physical Plant.*** Are the facilities modern or old? Have renovations been carried out as needed? Are renovations presently under way or contemplated? When was the institution established? Does it still occupy its original site? Is the agency housed in scattered, low-rise buildings or in a vertical, high-rise structure? Is the equipment modern or outdated?

• ***Ownership.*** Is the agency a for-profit or a not-for-profit institution? Is it freestanding or part of a conglomerate or consortium? Is it operated by the government or is it a private, voluntary institution?

• ***History.*** Have there been any changes in ownership of the agency? What was its original purpose or mission? Has there been any change in that mission?

• ***Reimbursement.*** What are the reimbursement sources of the agency and what is the proportion of each in its total revenues? Has the agency experienced problems with its reimbursement arrangements?

• ***Community Relations.*** What is the reputation of the agency within the community? Does the agency draw from the community for its patient base? for its personnel?

External Environment

• ***Community.*** Is the community an old, established one or has it grown up relatively recently? Is it predominantly rich, poor, or middle-class, or a mix? Is there a dominant ethnic group or religious affiliation? Is the community economically diversified or is it a "one-industry town"? If the latter, what type of industry?

• ***Competition.*** What other facilities of the same type are located nearby? What is the agency's marketing stance toward its competition?

Internal Environment

• ***Culture and Norms.*** What is the dominant communication style among personnel? On what basis are individuals rewarded? What do people get promoted for? What is the mix of professional versus nonprofessional staff? Is there any predominant ethnic or religious group? What metaphors are used within the institution to describe it? Has there been a change in culture or norms in the history of the agency? If so, when and why? Do subcultures exist in nursing or in other areas? Is there a formal dress code? Are the rules and policies of the institution rigid or flexible? What rites and rituals exist and what are the risks of not observing them?

• ***Organizational Structure.*** Is management structured on a centralized or decentralized basis, or is it a mix? What are the usual patterns of communication: top-down, bottom-up, rumor? Is management means- or ends-oriented?

• ***Personnel.*** Does the agency recruit professionally educated staff? Does it provide adequate on-the-job training or are new personnel thrown in and expected to sink or swim? Are employees encouraged to be people-oriented or task-oriented? Is money allocated to send staff to professional conferences or other outside activities? If so, is the money equally distributed? Are employees treated paternalistically or as adults? Are employees unionized or in the process of unionizing?

• ***Management Style.*** Is management participative, authoritarian, flexible, or a mix? Do managers observe an open-door policy with subordinates? Is empire building important? Is performance or politics more important? Is information readily available to all or is it "top secret"?

Principal Players and Supporting Characters

• ***Characteristics.*** For each participant in the story: What is his or her age, sex, ethnic and/or religious background? How long has he or she been in the job? How did this individual get there? Is he or she an old-timer who has come up through the ranks? a newcomer brought in from outside? a fast-tracker? a favorite son or protege? Is this individual's strong suit administrative or technical competence or political savvy? Is his or her status maintained by credentials, high visibility, or personal credibility?

• ***Relationships.*** What are the formal and informal relationships among and between the characters in the story? What are their vested interests and hidden agendas?

Background

What significant events, external and internal, preceded the story told here? Were there reimbursement changes, economic climate changes, changes in ownership or administration, changes in values or culture? How is the nursing department characterized? What is its size? its personnel mix? its delivery system? its practice emphasis? What is its attitude toward innovation? Who in the department are "organization people" and who are "outsiders"? What kind of rapport exists between nursing and the attending physicians at the institution? What is the department's organizational structure? Is there collective bargaining with management? How do such things as office location, allocation of resources and space, committee membership, and job titles reflect the status of nursing at the institution?

case analysis

Friends in high places

Relevant Information

Norms, Values, Sacred Cows

- Appearances are important; the physical appearance of the hospital is cheerful and homey; patient complaints of rudeness elicited major educational efforts.
- Board of Trustees members hold power through long-term inherited appointment to the Board. They are all women because of the hospital's original mission.
- "Ownership" of the hospital is a very personal issue with members of the Board, particularly the COB.
- The ethnic composition of hospital administration does not match that of the external environment.
- Promotion and rewards are related to belonging to the right groups.
- Management style is avoidance.

Relationships and Power Needs

- The DON is very cognizant of the values of the Board of Trustees and caters to their needs, particularly the COB's. The DON knows "her place."
- The DON has no budgetary decision power and therefore must play games to get what she wants.

• Staff are kept ignorant of what goes on both inside and in the outside world. This may be a means of control. Their frustration has created union activity among the ranks.

• The Board makes many operational decisions.

• The nursing organizational chart shows a traditional line structure with multiple layers of management, all of whom have minimal authority.

• The COB, extremely wealthy, has many political connections which she uses to keep the hospital in business.

• The CMS and the ADSD are professional allies.

Hidden Agendas and Vested Interests

• Quality of care is a professed objective of the new ADSD, an outsider in her first top management job.

• Innovation and change are the interest of some; others are interested in maintaining the status quo.

• The ADSD perceives the DON's noninterference to be approval of her prior activities, most of which were essential to meet accreditation requirements.

Answers to Questions

1. Success for this DON was her tenure in the position in the face of documented declining quality of nursing care. Reviewing the norms and values of the organization, it is clear that maintaining appearances and the status quo is more important than innovation and change. DON is also very savvy about where power resides. She recognizes the Chairman of the Board and other members as having ultimate power and maintains the correct relationships with these individuals. DON has seen others come and go, she recognizes and conforms to the established values of the organization. She fosters personal relationships and does not attempt to grasp authority or power for herself, but rather uses others' power and authority to her advantage. She will probably remain in this position until she is ready to retire.

2. Unlike the DON, these two players are both politically naive. They believe in competent performance and did not tune in to the real messages related to organizational norms and values.

The ASDN may not have done an adequate assessment of the organization before taking the job. A careful scrutiny of staffing, past practices, and the lack of previous educational activities may have alerted her to the probability of success of any changes. Her naivete and lack of experience may have precluded her awareness of the true power relationships and individual goals.

The CMS, also an outsider, like the ADSD did not look at the context in which the clinical problems were occurring. The CMS and the ADSD might have formed a coalition with the assistant hospital administrator. This individual controlled the daily operational decisions, appeared to be interested in performance, and may have been willing to help them. By going to the DON and the HA, the CMS put both of them in a position of confrontation, an uncomfortable and atypical situation for both. As could have been predicted, nothing was done, life went on, and the individuals who wouldn't or couldn't recognize and manage the cultural norms and power relationships retreated from the field. Success is in survival.

case analysis

Vested interests

RELEVANT INFORMATION

Norms, Values, Sacred Cows

- The hospital is located in a traditional community with a single dominant religious affiliation and strong labor sympathies among the permanent residents.
- Both the HA and the DON belong to religious groups different from the norm.
- Physicians are the elitists both in the hospital and in the community.
- Hospital staff resisted efforts to create rituals within the organization and to participate in a "family" culture.
- There is a distinct barrier between regular residents and "touristas" and between old-timers and newcomers.
- The DON is a well-educated single woman, different from the norm for women her age in the hospital and in the community.
- The "new breed" of nurses has different values from the old guard.

Relationships and Power Needs

- A threat of financial collapse stimulated action on the part of the Board. After seven years of new management, the financial situation is excellent.

• The Board is dominated by physicians and local old-timers.

• New comers and touristas have no power in decision making in the community.

• Old-timers have no power in the hospital since the management change seven years ago.

• Three departments were dropped down a notch in the new organizational structure.

• The HA and the DON are a strong support team and often form a triangle with the Staff Radiologist and other physicians.

• The HA took some decision-making power away from the Board.

• The Director of Personnel has strong ties to the community and Board members.

• There are physicians' assistants but no nurse practitioners in the community.

Hidden Agendas and Vested Interests

• The Staff Radiologist, an old-timer in the community, has power and control needs beyond what is vested in his formal position.

• The Director of Mental Health, a spy in the organization, was demoted in the reporting hierarchy in the change but still has access to privileged information.

• Old-guard nurses are not career oriented, but need their jobs for financial security.

• Physicians assert their power by negotiating with the striking nurses even though it is in defiance of labor laws and formal authority rules.

Answers to Questions

1. The poststrike status of individuals and departments can be explained by an analysis of the interaction of power and status needs in a changing economic climate. Physicians, who saw their power diminished by the actions of the Board and the new administrator, took advantage of the strike opportunity to seize back power. The Director of Mental Health, who aligned himself with the physicians, gained in status and authority. The Staff Radiologist is more powerful as a result of his promotion to Chief of Medical Staff. The Director of Personnel remains, although in a lower hierarchical position, not because of competence but because of his strong social and blood connections.

The Assistant Director of Education, closely identified with the DON, resigned upon recognizing her probable termination or reassignment. Social Service has been elevated in the reporting hierarchy, another dilution of the nursing department's power base. The Director of Finance, although hired originally by the HA, remains, probably because of his knowledge of the hospital's financial picture. His future success will depend on relationships with the new administrator.

2. The situation as reported resulted partially from the failure of the HA and the DON to assess accurately the power needs of physicians and the importance of cultural norms in this setting. No doubt both of these individuals would have been more successful and survived in the system had their "sins" been singular. However, the combination of ignorance of the proper place of women and nurses, irreverence for physicians, religious differences, and changes in the value/reward system was collectively too much to be tolerated. There was probably also jealousy of the HA's ability to mount and implement programs that successfully competed with the nearby big city hospitals. If the DON had compromised her philosophy and formed alliances with a few powerful physicians, her termination might have been prevented. Power struggles might have been negotiated or in some cases, such as reopening beds after the strike, been conceded.

Some organizational theorists believe that organizations, like individuals and groups, proceed through developmental stages such as cohesion, trust building, innovation, creativity, and autonomy. Progression through these stages is not necessarily linear nor always desirable. This case study seems to illustrate a situation in which innovation and creativity which led to hospital-wide improvement were not sufficient to overcome group norms and power needs, which culminated in a return after the strike to a traditional organizational structure and power base.

3. The future of the department of nursing is rather easy to predict. The new DON will be selected on the basis of her ability to work within the traditions of the hospital and community culture. The new breed of nurses will be tolerated only as long as positions need to be filled, but they will not be encouraged. The union may eventually be decertified, but while it exists it will certainly be weak because of its open-shop base. Negotiation of future contracts will probably be pro forma, with management offers being accepted with little discussion.

It is likely that a similar cycle of events will occur if the physicians' need for control conflicts with the hospital administration's need to maintain financial stability, and vested interests will continue to be powerful in influencing future events.

case analysis

The politics of illusion

Relevant Information

Norms, Values, Sacred Cows

• The traditional values of the organization are being challenged by the newcomers.

• Two incongruent cultures are operating simultaneously. One stresses maintaining the status quo, while the other emphasizes productivity and accountability.

• The new image desired by the newcomers is one that may be perceived as alienating and a put-down to the old-timers.

• The reward system has been changed.

• In the nursing department, confrontation is being encouraged, another contradiction to the previous norm, "Let sleeping dogs lie."

• Drawing attention to the differences between reality and hope or illusion is not appreciated--this norm, however, is one the DON ignores and contradicts.

Relationships and Power Needs

• Although governance has changed, real power is still vested in the Board, which is controlled by politicians and local industry executives.

• Culture and gender relationships are strained and unequal in their access to power.

• Informal relationships based on culture, gender, and position that were successful in the past have been devalued by the newcomers.

• Authority is being decentralized in the nursing department, a break with tradition and former relationships.

• The DON has not established ties or contacts within the community or with the Board members.

• Management style is inconsistent in the newcomer group.

• Informal strong relationships exist between some of the principal players.

• Titles do not necessarily reflect real power or ability to make things happen.

• The HA is very sensitive to the relative status of physicians and administrators.

• Authority and power are not vested in the same individuals.

• The dress code committee's recommendations are overruled and become a *cause celebre*.

• Many organizational decisions are made outside the formal structure.

Hidden Agendas and Vested Interests

• The hospital is used as a political football by would-be office seekers.

• Empire building is too important to many of the newcomers.

• Opportunity to add experience to professional resumes is a vested interest for several administrators.

• The CMS failed once in a previous administrative role and now needs to prove himself as well as to enhance his reputation and status in the medical school.

- The CEO is marking time.
- The HA wants the ADN out of the organization.

Answers to Questions

1. Ultimately, the physicians won the struggle over the obstetrical service brouhaha. Although some of the nursing staff did document unacceptable behaviors displayed by resident physicians, most of the nurses were reluctant to follow through with documentation or formal complaints. When the DON left, conditions reverted to what they had been. Several RNs then also left.

2. All of the newcomers ultimately left the organization. The DON resigned out of frustration, the CEO found another high-level post in the government, the HA was forced to resign when he began to hold people accountable, and the assistant administrators went on to bigger and better opportunities.

A new DON has been hired and the old-guard players are still in place. The ADN is still there and continues in the good graces of those in power.

3. (See relevant information).

4. The factors that may explain the ultimate outcomes in this case are as follows:

a. The DON's style and values were incongruent with the organization's personality. She did not conform with either the old-guard's norms or the new-guard's illusions. She also failed to establish a support base with community leaders or Board members.

b. Power plays and vested interests, not quality of care, were the real issues for several principal players.

c. Maintenance was a greater driving force than innovation in this organization. It is unlikely that the client base or hospital image will change. This hospital will probably always be perceived and identified as the "county" hospital in spite of new facades and a new name. Old wine, new label--no real change.

case analysis

Complex relationships

RELEVANT INFORMATION

Norms, Values, Sacred Cows

- Parent-child relationships set the tone for interactions between employees and management.
- A strong organizational culture based on shared ethnic beliefs and values leads to intolerance and mistrust of outsiders.
- Longevity and loyalty to the organization are rewarded, often without regard to performance.
- Norms of mediocrity and preservation of the status quo prevail throughout the organization.
- Middle management in the nursing department is restrictive and punitive.
- Norms of the past are being challenged by the vice-president for nursing:
    - management style is changing from authoritarian to participative;
    - new leadership has been brought in from the outside rather than promoted from within;
    - new programs and policies are changing the status quo.

Relationships and Power Needs

• Informal power derives from favorable status with the nuns.

• The Vice-President for Financial Services has greater power than that associated with the position; as mother superior of the local order, plans are run by her for approval.

• The order of nuns still retains ultimate power, although this was challenged somewhat by the medical staff's ouster of the nun-administrator five years ago.

• Both the President and the VPN will be more vulnerable to the whims and desires of the nuns because the hospital will not renew its contract with the national management corporation.

• The DNP has the power to hold the VPN hostage because of her favored status with the nuns.

• The first Director of Nursing continues to yield influence among nursing staff by her constant interaction with the staff.

Hidden Agendas and Vested Interests

• All persons in administrative positions have a stake in keeping on the "good side" of the nuns.

• Two vice-presidents (for professional services and planning and development) have vested interests in turf-building in order to compensate for their incompetence.

• The DNP could subvert the nursing vice-president's new directions and plans.

Answers to Questions

1. If the VPN fires the DNP, she can hire someone whose philosophy and management style is consistent with her own. However, firing the DNP would violate the organization's cultural norms of longevity and loyalty. If the VPN moves the DNP into another position, she may reduce the DNP's positional power, but the DNP may still have influence among the nursing staff.

2. The VPN did discuss the DNP situation with the influential nuns. The VPN was careful not to seek their permission for her contemplated action, but she did get a feel for their support for her, even if she would fire the DNP.

case analysis

A fatal attack

Relevant Information

Norms, Values, Sacred Cows

• The hospital is proud to be considered the leading hospital in the city and of its position as a provider of community services in addition to health care.

• There is an old guard composed of established residents who have a WASP culture and are old-money or tradespeople. The newcomers are welcome but not considered part of the "in" group.

• Rituals and formality are important, and taking part in the rituals is expected.

• A family metaphor is used in describing the hospital.

• The DON is a newcomer and a member of a different religious group.

• Status symbols are not overt--everyone is supposed to know who is important.

• Wives of important men have influence on what happens in the community.

Relationships and Power Needs

• Although a family atmosphere is touted, everyone in the hospital is supposed to know his or her place.

- The top two administrative positions are filled by "good old boys" or old-guard members.
- The AA is put out by the fact that the DON reports to the CEO instead of to himself.
- The AA is ambitious.
- The AA is married to the director of the hospital's LPN program.
- The DON is popular and also ambitious.
- The DON is married to the DMS, who is very powerful and beloved.
- The DMS and the CEO are friends.
- The DMS indulges his wife, a practice resented by a number of people.
- The CS and the AA have formed an alliance both in the hospital and socially.
- The DON is a voting member of several medical board committees.

Hidden Agendas and Vested Interests

- The AA believes the organization needs more control and a tighter structure.
- The CS thinks nurses should be kept in their place. He will be the DMS's successor.
- The director of the LPN program, married to the AA, does not approve of the DON.
- The DON wants to change the staffing mix to increase RN positions and reduce LPN positions.
- Most physicians don't want any nurse to be a voting member of medical board committees.

Answers to Questions

1. Prior to the Director of Medical Staff's death, the proposal had an excellent chance of being approved. The plan was sup-

ported by the CEO as it touched on one of his vested interests, patient education; it would continue positive relationships with the community; and it would be no more costly than previous staffing plans. The DON had also gotten support from the nursing practice council and from the younger LPN staff. The DON's husband, a voting member of the Board of Trustees, had also agreed to use his very considerable influence over other trustees. With the death of the DMS, the probability of success decreases dramatically. The Board of Trustees may very well postpone the board meeting out of respect for the DMS. Valuable time and momentum may be lost, and in the interim the physicians and their wives who are not enamored of the DON may exert their influence to oppose the plan. The AA and his wife, who of course will lose her position as director of the LPN program if the plan is implemented, will certainly exert their influence to oppose the plan. The DON, however, may also use the sympathy and positive feelings toward her deceased husband to pressure the Board of Trustee members.

(Note: In the actual case, the DON issued an immediate plea through a handwritten note to all board members requesting they honor her husband's desire to see this plan through and also requested they establish a memorial scholarship fund in his name to support a specific number of LPN staff to further their education via the ADN program. This strategy was successful in saving her proposal, which was approved with a few modifications relating to phase-out time for the LPN school.)

2. The DON's immediate future seems secure. However, since the CEO is retiring in two years, probably to be succeeded by the AA, no friend to the DON, she may not have long-term tenure in the position. She can either use the two years to wield influence toward getting an outside successor to the CEO or look for another position.

Although the DON was a very successful strategist and a competent director, she did alienate a number of the old guard as well as several powerful physicians. The probability of her turning around these negative feelings is minimal. Therefore, she may be wiser to leave while she is still "on top."

PART IV

Readings on Power and Politics in Organizations

How to Swim with Sharks: A Primer

BY VOLTAIRE COUSTEAU*

Actually, nobody *wants* to swim with sharks. It is not an acknowledged sport, and it is neither enjoyable nor exhilarating. These instructions are written primarily for the benefit of those who, by virtue of their occupation, find they *must* swim and find that the water is infested with sharks.

Swimming with sharks is like any other skill: it cannot be learned from books alone; the novice must practice in order to develop the skill. The following rules simply set forth the fundamental principles which, if followed, will make it possible to survive while becoming expert through practice.

Rule 1. **Assume unidentified fish are sharks.** Not all sharks look like sharks, and some fish which are not sharks sometimes act like sharks. Unless you have witnessed docile behavior in the presence of shed blood on more than one occasion, it is best to assume an unknown species is a shark.

* Little is known about the author, who died in Paris in 1812. He may have been a descendant of Francois Voltaire and an ancestor of Jacques Cousteau. Apparently this essay was written for sponge divers. Because it may have broader implications, it was translated from the French by Richard J. Johns, an obscure French scholar and Massey Professor and director of the Department of Biomedical Engineering, The Johns Hopkins University and Hospital, 720 Rutland Avenue, Baltimore, Maryland 21205.

Rule 2. **Do not bleed.** It is a cardinal principle that if you are injured either by accident or by intent you must not bleed. Experience shows that bleeding prompts an even more aggressive attack.

Admittedly, it is difficult not to bleed when injured. Indeed, at first this may seem impossible. Diligent practice, however, will permit the experienced swimmer to sustain a serious laceration without bleeding and without even exhibiting any loss of composure. This hemostatic reflex can in part be conditioned, but there may be constitutional aspects as well. Those who cannot learn to control their bleeding should not attempt to swim with sharks, for the peril is too great.

The control of bleeding has a positive protective element for the swimmer. The shark will be confused as to whether or not his attack has injured you, and confusion is to the swimmer's advantage. On the other hand, the shark may know he has injured you and be puzzled as to why you do not bleed or show distress. This also has a profound effect on sharks. They begin questioning their own potency or, alternatively, believe the swimmer to have supernatural powers.

Rule 3. **Counter any aggression promptly.** Sharks rarely attack a swimmer without warning. Usually there is some tentative, exploratory aggressive action. It is important that the swimmer recognizes that this behavior is a prelude to an attack and takes prompt and vigorous remedial action. The appropriate countermove is a sharp blow to the nose. Almost invariably this will prevent a full-scale attack, for it makes it clear that you understand the shark's intentions and are prepared to use whatever force is necessary to repel his aggressive actions.

Some swimmers mistakenly believe that an ingratiating attitude will dispel an attack under these circumstances. This is not correct; such a response provokes a shark attack. Those who hold this erroneous view can usually be identified by their missing limb.

Rule 4. **Get out if someone is bleeding.** If a swimmer (or shark) has been injured and is bleeding, get out of the water promptly. The presence of blood and the thrashing of water will elicit aggressive behavior even in the most docile of sharks. This latter group, poorly skilled in attacking, often behaves irrationally and may attack uninvolved swimmers or sharks. Some are so inept that in the confusion they injure themselves.

No useful purpose is served in attempting to rescue the injured swimmer. He either will or will not survive the attack, and your intervention cannot protect him once blood has been shed.

Rule 5. **Use anticipatory retaliation.** A constant danger to the skilled swimmer is that the sharks will forget that he is skilled and may attack in error. Some sharks have notoriously poor memories in this regard. This memory loss can be prevented by a program of anticipatory retaliation. The skilled swimmer should engage in these activities periodically, and the periods should be less than the memory span of the shark. Thus, it is not possible to state fixed intervals. The procedure may need to be repeated frequently with forgetful sharks and need be done only once for sharks with total recall.

The procedure is essentially the same as described under rule 3--a sharp blow to the nose. Here, however, the blow is unexpected and serves to remind the shark that you are both alert and unafraid. Swimmers should take care not to injure the shark and draw blood during this exercise for two reasons: First, sharks often bleed profusely, and this leads to the chaotic situation described under rule 4. Second, if swimmers act in this fashion it may not be possible to distinguish swimmers from sharks.

Rule 6. **Disorganize an organized attack.** Usually sharks are sufficiently self-centered that they do not act in concert against a swimmer. This lack of organization greatly reduces the risk of swimming among sharks. However, upon occasion the sharks may launch a coordinated attack upon a swimmer or even upon one of their number.

The proper strategy is diversion. Sharks can be diverted from their organized attack in one of two ways. First, sharks as a group are especially prone to internal dissension. An experienced swimmer can divert an organized attack by introducing something, often something minor or trivial, which sets the sharks to fighting among themselves. Usually by the time the internal conflict is settled the sharks cannot even recall what they were setting about to do,much less get organized to do it.

A second mechanism of diversion is to introduce something which so enrages the members of the group that they begin to lash out in all directions, even attacking inanimate objects in their fury.

What should be introduced? Unfortunately, different things prompt internal dissension or blind fury in different groups of sharks. Here one must be experienced in dealing with a given group of sharks, for what enrages one group will pass unnoted by another.

It is scarcely necessary to state that it is unethical for a swimmer under attack by a group of sharks to counter the attack by diverting them to another swimmer. It is, however, common to see this done by novice swimmers and by sharks when they fall under a concerted attack.

A Model for Politically Astute Planning and Decision Making

Karen S. Ehrat

The administrative role in both nursing service and education demands many political interfaces that encompass conflicts, negotiations, power struggles and on-going competition for scarce resources. However, the skill required to deal effectively with those situations is a function of both career and organizational experiences. The model presented in this article is intended to provide nurse administrators with a framework for politically astute planning and decision making and avoidance of judgment faux pas.

The contemporary nursing administrative role, in both service and education, requires expertise that extends beyond the planning, budgeting, controlling, and other classical managerial functions. The role demands the ability to deal skillfully with the implicit and explicit variables the administrator confronts. Yet the acquisition of political skill is principally by rigorous and repeated trial and error across the span of a career. The conceptual model for political planning

---

Reprinted with permission from the *Journal of Nursing Administration* 13 (September 1983): 29-35.

and decision making presented here is intended to reduce the error in that process and to assist the novice manager to avoid political pitfalls. A situational application of the model is provided to lend clarity.

Throughout the discussion, the reader should recognize that becoming more political in method does not mean becoming more politicized in the sense of having an ideological basis for decision[1]. Behaving politically implies neither irresponsibility nor insensitivity. Rather, it involves the meshing of sound strategy with individual values and ethics.

Politics is the art of getting what one wants within the totality of complex organizational relationships--using the ability to manipulate the variables to one's favor or advantage. Manipulation in this instance refers to the skillful and artistic management of available resources. It is the ability to gain more influence than others, utilizing the same resources[2].

In any instance where authority and power exists, a political climate prevails. Politics is the nature of human society. Our own society is founded on the idea of democracy, and democracy is a political process. The democratic process is an arena of compromise, trade-offs, favors, and negotiations. Taken as a whole, the system is highly efficient because only a few issues are of importance to any one interest group (save catastrophic events). By and large, the numerous and various special interest groups are willing to negotiate and compromise to satisfy their particular interests. Not unlike the fundamental and founding idea of democracy, management is a process of compromise, negotiations, and trade-offs. Given that nursing is interdependent in an organizational sense, nurse managers must be equipped to negotiate and compromise for the overall welfare of nursing and patient care.

Effective political behavior cannot be prescribed, for what will be effective depends on the situation--the issue at hand, the cast, the players, the stakes, and the potential gains to be acquired. Instead, effective political behavior results from careful consideration of the multiple forces in operation. The following model represents a distillation of organizational dynamics and social forces into various fundamental political concepts that impinge upon managerial effectiveness.

The Model

Exhibit 1 depicts continuums of structure, economy, process, and outcome that need consideration and careful juxtaposition in the planning and decision-making process. The model is not intended to be prescriptive but is a schematic guidepost to facilitate the identification of political interfaces. Each concept will be discussed independently, though it is recognized that many of the concepts interrelate.

Structure Considerations

Idiosyncracies of an organization make it a unique entity. The structure considerations that contribute to that uniqueness include organizational history, the budget operation, and data deemed administratively to be significant.

History. One of the most important political concepts is history. From the plethora of literature addressing change theory and change strategies, one can assume that organizations or institutions are run largely on the basis of past experiences. History and tradition, as well as market forces, appear to be the major shaping forces of most organizations. Except in crisis or major administrative transition, organizations are unlikely to change dramatically, owing to their resistive natures. Schon notes that crisis and disruption are required to break the stable state of organizations[3].

Similarly, individuals operate from an experiential or historical base and, to one degree or another, struggle to preserve the norm. Lawrence and Allan believe that five sources of information affect organizational policy decisions: in order of priority they are personal experience (history), constituents, organized pressure groups, media, and research (factual data)[4]. Certain of these factors may influence operational as well as in-

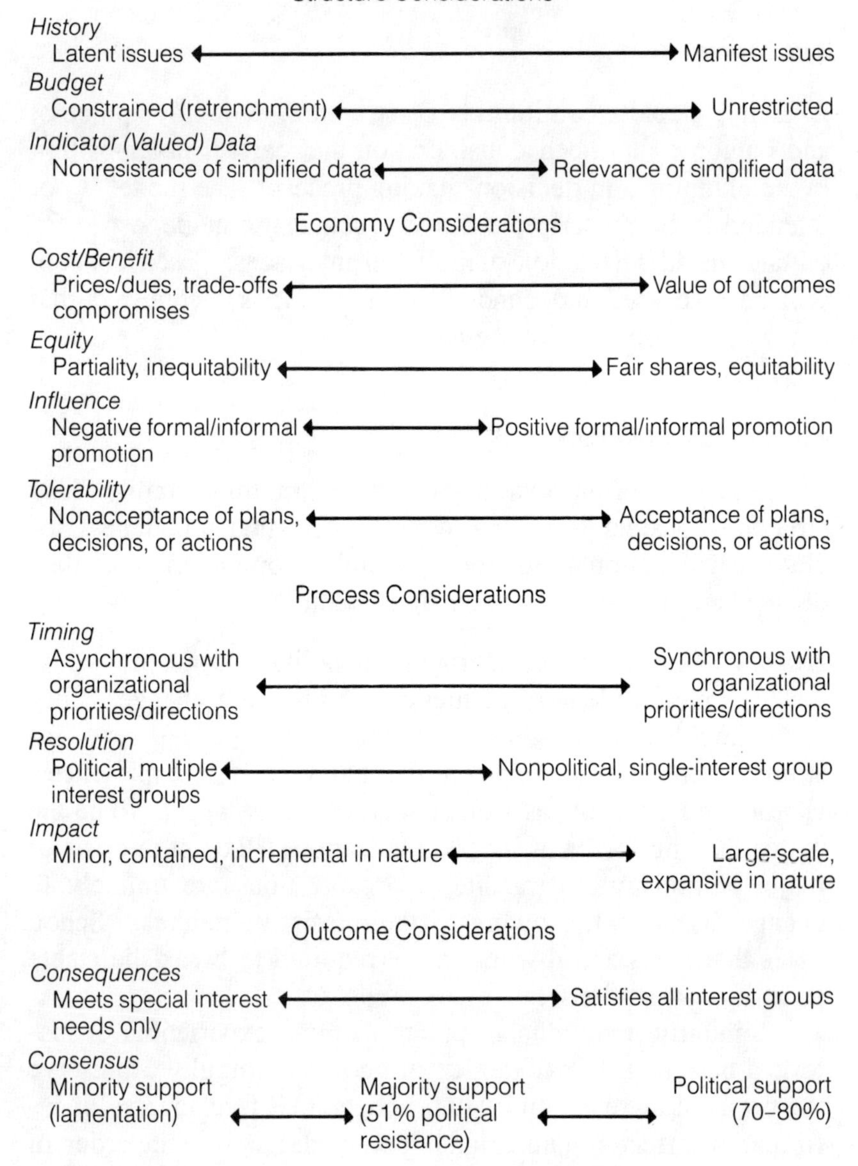
EXHIBIT 1.
MODEL OF POLITICAL INTERFACES
Structure Considerations
History
Latent issues
Manifest issues
Budget
Constrained (retrenchment)
Unrestricted
Indicator (Valued) Data
Nonresistance of simplified data
Relevance of simplified data
Economy Considerations
Cost/Benefit
Prices/dues, trade-offs compromises
Value of outcomes
Equity
Partiality, inequitability
Fair shares, equitability
Influence
Negative formal/informal promotion
Positive formal/informal promotion
Tolerability
Nonacceptance of plans, decisions, or actions
Acceptance of plans, decisions, or actions
Process Considerations
Timing
Asynchronous with organizational priorities/directions
Synchronous with organizational priorities/directions
Resolution
Political, multiple interest groups
Nonpolitical, single-interest group
Impact
Minor, contained, incremental in nature
Large-scale, expansive in nature
Outcome Considerations
Consequences
Meets special interest needs only
Satisfies all interest groups
Consensus
Minority support (lamentation)
Majority support (51% political resistance)
Political support (70–80%)

dividual decisions. Presumably organizational norms and priorities are the way they are for reasons that may be latent. Thus gaining a perspective on the latent issues prior to making a decision or taking action seems worthwhile. In other words one must have an understanding of the past in order to deal skillfully with the present.

Virtually every major issue that an organization confronts has a history. It has been suggested that those issues revolve in some timed fashion along a carousel course. With respect to administrative priorities, a revolving pattern may also be evident in the past nature of the organization. Efforts toward effective and successful planning and decision making are facilitated by a working knowledge of past struggles and outcomes.

Budget. A second major political concept is budgeting. The budget has been said to be a representation of organizational activity in monetary terms. The budget accurately reflects the outcomes of the previous year's political struggles. Generally, the budgetary process operates on a zero sum principle, a finite set of resources irrespective of allocation demands. In most situations, new resource allocations come at the expense or demise of presently funded programs or departments. Thus the processes of negotiations, trade-offs, and compromises come into play. When the economy is constrained and budget costs seem necessary, it is a foregone conclusion that the cutting of resources or personnel forces institutional efficiency and increases productivity. Managers tend to react by trying to protect their vested interests by whatever means possible.

Prior to any final decision the manager should consider the impact of the decision on the budget and should recognize that any attempt at change will draw administrative and organizational attention. The manager's vested interests pass before the reviewing stand and may be subject to budgetary constriction by higher authority. If cost savings or efficiency can be built into the decision package, the decision is less likely to meet organized resistance. Note too that in times of economic scarcity political activity increases as individuals or departments compete for declining resources.

Indicator (Valued) Data

Organizations are to one degree or another simplified. Owing to the breadth and complexity of organizational activity, it is impossible for any one individual to have an in-depth understanding of each organizational department or unit. Wildavsky notes that one method for handling complexity is to use simpler items as indices of more complicated ones[5]. Within organizations key administrative personnel utilize certain simple indicators to monitor and evaluate the welfare of the whole, a system of checks and balances. Regarding the status of employee safety, for example, appropriate simple indicators might be the number and dollar amounts of workman compensation claims rather than individual employee injuries. Likewise, to assess the overall attitude or morale in nursing, the administrator might look at turnover rates, sick-absent statistics, labor activity, and so forth. Assumptions are made about the whole based on certain simple indicators. Those key, but arbitrary, parameters provide administrative personnel with a fundamental mechanism for evaluating and making judgments about the organization. But minor aberrations are obscured by the whole.

With respect to nursing management and decision making, managers should familiarize themselves with indicator data valued by the organization and monitor it rigorously. Familiarity with institutional history and present-day labor and financial trends will help in identifying those important indicators. Any significant change in that indicator data should cue the manager to take a proactive rather than a reactive course of planning and action. An overview of any corrective action should be directed administratively. Unrelated nursing decisions and actions are advanced with less administrative resistance when valued nursing indicator data are kept within the parameters deemed acceptable by the administrator.

Economy Considerations

Economy considerations have to do with weighing the cost versus the benefit and the risk versus the expected outcomes or potential consequences in any given situation. In all noncrisis planning and decision-making processes, it is vital to devote sufficient energy to economy concerns. There is a point beyond which the probable consequences outweigh the gains to be realized.

Cost/Benefit. Another concept worth singling out of the political milieu is the notion of prices or dues. Payment is required for whatever one achieves, regardless of the worth or merit of the achievement itself. There are dues to pay, trade-offs to be made, and compromises to effect. Only the buyer can determine when the stakes are too high or when his or her personal values are overly compromised. The issue is basically one of economics: cost versus benefit. The costs may be either explicit or implicit in nature. What does one have to gain and what is the actual price or potential price?

Within an organizational network, it is politically naive not to consider the issues of price and dues in the planning process. Every successful gain that is achieved in a political environment has its consequences. It is the degree of those consequences that the nursing manager must attempt to predict and evaluate. When a gain in nursing compromises another discipline or department or results in the perception of inequitable treatment, the stakes must be carefully considered. It has been suggested that within organizations friends or supporters come and go depending on what is to be gained by them, but enemies or nonsupporters tend to accumulate over time. There are some battles to be lost in the long-range interest of winning the war.

Equity. Another political concept that relates in some fashion to budget has to do with fair shares and equity. Each department or organizational division expects to receive the budget allocation that it received last year plus its fair share of funds over and above last year's budget[6]. Similarly, in years of budgetary cutbacks, each department expects to be affected only to the extent that other departments are affected. In the end and from an administrative view, all things (particularly with reference to monies allocated) must be fair and equitable rather than arbitrary. Thus any plan for nursing change that demands more resources than deemed equitable by top administration is likely to fail. Because it is more or less assumed by all parties involved that a privilege once extended becomes a right, few arbitrary judgments are likely to be made with respect to resource allocations.

Influence. Another economy consideration in planning and decision making is influence. When political situations are at hand, careful thought must be given to who best can introduce and successfully sell the decision or plan to those concerned. A person's influence is perceived by others when that person exercises political savvy, has developed a clientele, is confident, has a meaningful network, has administrative support, exercises effective platform skills, and exploits available opportunity. It entails the skillful utilization and manipulation of the multiple resources at the person's disposal and the application of personal strengths, expertise, and knowledge to any given situation. The exercise of influence is a critical factor in any successful nursing maneuver. Therefore, when advancing nursing reform in a political environment, it may be to the advantage of that reform effort if the promoters are perceived by the organization as having positive influence and can exercise that influence unobtrusively[7].

Tolerability. It appears to be reasonable to acknowledge that organizations issue new managers or administrators complementary, though hypothetical, "limb" (out-on-a-limb) passes, number and expiration unknown. If used, these passes are reserved for situations where conviction compels action without regard for political risk and consequences. Related to limb passes is the political concept of tolerability, or limits of tolerance. In any given organization and situation, there are ill-de-

EXHIBIT 2.
ALGORITHM FOR DETERMINING THE
LIMITS OF TOLERABILITY

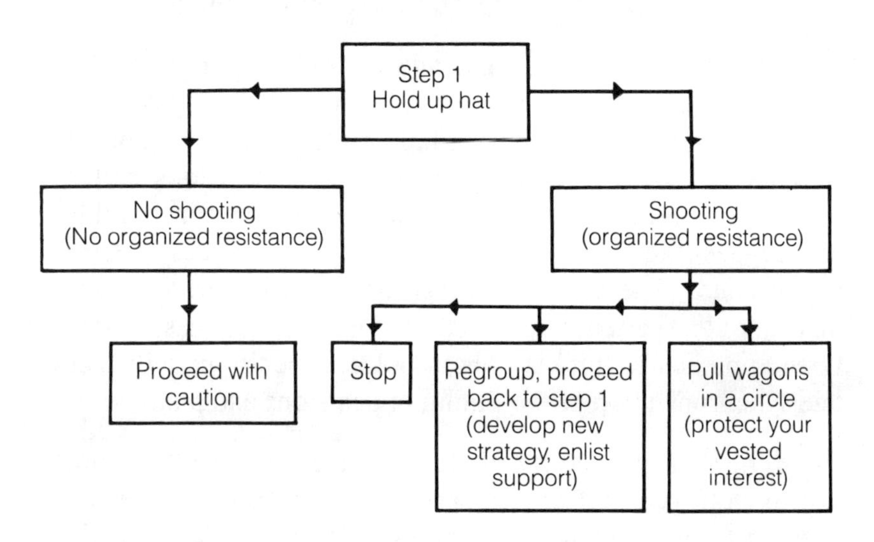

fined limits or boundaries of tolerance beyond which behavior, decisions, or actions will not be accepted, and beyond which consequences will follow. Despite their lack of clarity, these limits are not necessarily arbitrary but more probably relate to historical artifact within the organization. Thus in the planning process the politically rational behavior commands you to hold up your hat to see who is shooting before pursuing major actions, as is illustrated by the tongue-in-cheek algorithm shown in Exhibit 2. It is suggested that any action, decision, or proposed change that denies or ignores the realities of existing power, influence, and authority is probably too naive to be practical and most likely will not be tolerated.

Process Considerations

Yet another set of conceptual abstractions concerns the process of making a decision and implementing it. The intent is that these and other considerations will guide the manager in more thorough and thoughtful planning and decision making. Process considerations force the manager to think through the decision and its potential impact prior to implementation.

Timing. Most successful managers would agree that every idea, plan, decision, and action has its time. If timing is gauged inaccurately, the best laid plans fail. Unfortunately no concrete formula exists for evaluating the timing of decisions and actions. Consideration of the continuums presented in Exhibit 1 will suggest the appropriateness of timing regardless of the issue at hand. The ability to gauge timing is in part a factor of managerial experience and maturation. Nonetheless, a structured approach to thinking about political decisions will facilitate synchronization of the timing of decisions and plans.

Resolution. It is useful to understand the fundamental properties of both political and nonpolitical decisions to better conceptualize the probable resolution of any given plan of action. If a given situation involves only a single, narrow interest group, it may be possible to arrive at a nonpolitical decision that best fits the situation. A nonpolitical decision is reached by considering a problem on its own terms and by evaluating proposals according to how well they solve the problem[8]. The intent of rational action is to find the best possible (effective, efficient, and equitable) solution without regard for who makes, supports, or opposes it. Compromise is almost always irrational.

A political decision, on the other hand, involves multiple interest groups and is seldom made on the merits of a proposal, but always on who makes it and who opposes it[9]. Diesing points out that a course of action that corrects economic or social deficiencies but increases political difficulties should be rejected, while an action that contributes to political improvement is desirable even if it is not entirely sound from an economic or social standpoint[10]. In this instance, compromise is always a rational procedure, for compromise is the taproot of the political process.

As indicated at the outset, most situations that nurse managers confront are political in nature owing to the fact that nursing does not operate as an autonomous entity within an organization. That suggests that nursing managers seeking reform should be prepared to negotiate and compromise. In certain situations, more may be lost than gained, depending upon both the nature and scope of the opposing forces. In attempting to promote political decisions, both flexibility and neutrality must be exercised. When issues are being debated or lobbied, be sure to leave an escape route open for the opposing party or parties so they can save face. It should be recognized that political decisions are incremental in nature and are unlikely to meet the needs of all those concerned.

Impact. Thus attention is drawn to the potential impact of the decision and to the political concept of *incrementalism.* Organizations, departments, and other subunits evolve in an incremental or decremental (rather than a comprehensive) fashion, with only minor changes evidenced at any step along the way. A political check-and-balance system operates to preserve the norm. In noncrisis situations, organizations display an air of dynamic conservatism, political forces that function to resist change and maintain existing patterns of power and authority[11]. Change does not occur on its merits alone, for the merit of any proposed change or decision is a matter of political interpretation.

Promoters of change should recognize that organizations as well as individuals seek stability and the continuance of historical norms. Strategies must be utilized that advance the recognition of merit and introduce political reform. The process of making change involves building a clientele and gaining the trust and confidence of supporters; determining where the opposition lies, what the risks are, what the price is, and what the trade-offs are; and having a sense of timing so as to deal efficiently with those variables. Even when efforts are successful, change is incremental in nature because of uncontrolled variables that are political in nature. Opportunities for other than incremental change are greatest during times of uncertainty or perceived crisis.

The implication for nurse administrators or managers seems self-evident. Strategies that promote incremental or phased changes are more likely to be successful than large-scale attempts. In general, political boundaries will tolerate incremental changes. Decisions that call for large-scale reforms may be operationally successful if enacted through a series of well-planned and well-executed incremental phases, providing that critical attention is given to political variables along the way. Incremental planning is evidence of a well-thought-through political strategy.

Outcome Considerations

Outcome considerations have to do with decision and action consequences. To be viable, political decisions must address some of the needs of all concerned and must achieve political consensus.

Consequences. Administrative actions and decisions within organizations attempt to "*satisfice*" the needs and desires of all concerned personnel within the scope of available resources (the new word *satisfice* was invented to denote making a compromise between satisfying and sacrificing[12]). It is a foregone conclusion that all employees, physicians, contracted workers, and clientele will not be happy and their numerous diverse needs cannot be met. Administrators of health care organizations, like other business or corporate heads, therefore attempt to get by, to come out all right, to avoid trouble--to satisfice.

The concept of satisficing relates to economic scarcity but is also applicable to budgeting, personnel policies, staffing concerns, scheduling, and other organizational practices. As Simon has observed, since no one can possibly know all the alternatives and options of a given situation, a more reasonable model of decision making is to utilize limited information and resources to find solutions to problems that meet the minimum standards of satisfaction[13].

Health care organizations, like society, represent a maze of special interest groups lobbying for their respective causes. All interests and causes cannot be satisfied when the set of resources is finite and other organizational priorities and constraints exist. Thus the politically rational process is to attempt to "get by," to meet some of the desires of all concerned. Generally speaking, employees, physicians, and others will support decisions or proposals that meet at least some of their needs, on the principle that half a loaf is better than none.

The concept of satisficing has particular relevancy for nurse managers, since nursing directly interfaces with many other disciplines and ancillary workers. Most major nursing decisions have a certain amount of impact beyond the department of nursing. What is best for nursing may not be what is best or desired by other affected departments or personnel. Thus in the planning phase, efforts should be directed toward arriving at a decision that will satisfice, in some manner, the needs of all concerned. Evidence of efforts directed toward that end will positively affect the outcome. When such a decision cannot be effected, it is best to break down the plan of action into phases that can be enacted gradually and to prepare a strategy for dealing with resistance.

Consensus. The last political concept to be dealt with in the planning and decision-making model has to do with consensus. Despite the fact that the majority vote is the foundation on which a democratic society is built, justice is not necessarily done by going along with the majority. Political consensus is thought to be about 70 to 80 percent of the vote, compared to the 51 percent simple majority. Thus regardless of the fact that the numbers may favor a given line of thinking or action, they do not include the opposition. The strength of the opposition must be considered, and more important, the price to be paid for ignoring it. A decision or proposal that raises too many objections may in fact be a bad decision, or the timing of the decision may be wrong. The loudness of lamentation against the decision and the scope of the minority vote or opinion serve as reasonable indicators of the political milieu and further serve to predict the success of any given decision. With respect to major nursing decisions, certain compromises, trade-offs, or negotiations may have to be achieved to arrive at a political consensus.

Applying the Model

In order to appreciate fully the utility of the model presented in Exhibit 1, consider the example of a nurse administrator who desires to implement 10-hour shifts throughout the department of nursing.

Viewing the structure considerations first, an effort must be made to determine whether the hospital has traditionally dealt with shift alternatives. Equally important is whether key administrative personnel have had experience with such concepts; if so, it is critical to determine how they viewed those shift alternatives. Depending upon those historical facts, the administrator can better structure a plan and support for that plan.

Consideration must be given also to the broad budget picture, including patient revenues, cash flow, any efforts directed toward containing labor costs, and so forth. In an era of tight budgets and nursing salaries rising to meet the competition, it is unlikely that new dollars will be readily available. Hence the 10-hour shift proposal must be planned within the parameters of the existing nursing budget.

As noted earlier, various organizations value different types of indicator data. To be certain, all administrators are concerned with nursing turnover rates, new-hire costs (both recruitment and orientation), patient complaints, and physician dissatisfaction. Though these indicators may or may not relate to the 10-hour shift proposal, it behooves the nurse manager to have his or her house in order prior to advocating major change.

The other alternative is to make a case for how the 10-hour shift concept will improve those valued parameters.

Economy considerations then focus the manager toward issues of cost/benefit, equity, influence, and tolerability. Careful consideration must be given to both the cost and benefit of the 10-hour shift. One must attempt to determine both the financial outlays and other organizational costs. The probable reaction of ancillary departments must be considered, for instance. In order to gain the support or cooperation of those departments, thought must be given to the negotiations and trade-offs that will need to occur. Additionally, the effect of the 10-hour shift on overtime and education expenditures should be estimated. After thorough review of both the direct and indirect costs to nursing, the administrator must determine whether the gain to be made outweighs the cost.

Equity considerations are, at best, difficult to evaluate. If nursing implements 10-hour shifts in a full-scale manner, will ancillary services have the same opportunity? Or will resource allocations to nursing negatively impact allocations made to other service departments? Another consideration may be the hardships that 10-hour shifts in nursing pose for other departments. Clearly the answers to those questions are not universal but differ from one organization to another. But these issues must be thought through before proceeding forward. From an administrative view all choices must be equitable and fair rather than arbitrary. If equity cannot be demonstrated, perhaps a case can be made that cost savings or labor efficiency outweighs equity.

The nurse administrator who elects to go ahead with full-scale implementation of 10-hour shifts should determine in advance who can best lobby for this course in the organization. The person(s) selected must be able to exert influence positively, yet unobtrusively in order to move the organization toward the desired end. That person must also be willing and able to shoulder the responsibility should the plan fail.

It is always to the advantage of the manager to test the waters or gauge the limits of administrative tolerance before proceeding. In the example before us, perhaps the nurse administrators can through informal conversation pass before key administrators the thought that 10-hour shifts might improve financial concerns and patient outcomes. If the administrative response is other than purely negative, the decision maker can move forward in the planning process, exercising extreme caution. Conversely, if the response *is* negative, the decision maker should assume that the timing is wrong or that additional strategizing is necessary. Of course sometimes conviction compels action without regard for political risk and consequences. However high principled, such behavior is tolerated only up to a point though.

Process considerations look more closely at the issue of timing. If the timing of the 10-hour shift concept conflicts the priorities and directions of the organization can aid the decision maker in judging the best time to introduce or implement a plan or decision. Consideration of all continuums presented in Exhibit 1 will suggest the appropriate timing. If the timing of the 10-hour shift concept conflicts with other organizational priorities, a case might be made for the concept on the basis of cost effectiveness, reduction of nursing turnover, or other valid rationale. In other instances it may be more advisable and in the long run more successful to defer the plan until such time as it is more synchronous with organizational priorities.

Clearly the idea of the 10-hour shift is a political decision, for it involves, directly or indirectly, multiple interest groups. Political decisions call for first-hand attention to the prevention of discord and disruption. Since compromise is at the heart of the political process, the decision maker must be prepared to negotiate and compromise select aspects of the 10-hour shift plan. One such compromise might be agreement to pilot-test the plan in a confined area.

The impact of the implementation of the 10-hour shift throughout the department of nursing is clearly large scale, or expansive, in nature. No doubt less political resistance would ensue if the nurse administrator were to advocate an incremental approach--starting with thorough evaluation of the 10-hour shift on a single nursing unit before proceeding full scale, say. Again, lobbying for the whole to gain the part may be an effective strategy.

Looking at outcome considerations, certain negative consequences appear to be associated with full-scale implementation of 10-hour shifts throughout the department of nursing. Namely, the plan addressed special interest (nursing) needs only, ignoring all other service departments. To overcome or deal with that situation, a strategy that breaks the plan of action into incremental phases might be utilized. Further, certain of the political resistance might be allayed by incorporating certain ancillary service department managers in the evaluation process.

Finally, one must consider consensus. Regardless of the fact that the majority of nurses may favor 10-hour shifts, that support does not include the political opposition, both nursing and nonnursing. In this example proceeding slowly in an incremental fashion may help to dissipate or exhaust certain of the opposition. To be sure, nursing is unlikely to achieve political consensus unless the 10-hour shift can be demonstrated to benefit ancillary services.

In a situation where nursing strongly favors a given proposal (such as the 10-hour shift) but the political milieu contraindicates introduction of the plan, the nurse manager may buy time and continue to support the nursing interest by establishing a nursing committee or task force to research the concept further.

As can be gathered from this example, the model depicted in Exhibit 1 does not offer an exact prescription for political planning and decision making. Rather, it assists the manager to identify the many political issues that need consideration for successful decision making and planning in an organization.

Conclusion

The model for political planning and decision making presented in Exhibit 1 is not intended to represent the sum total of concerns that nurse managers must take into account in their decision processes. Rather, it is intended to serve as a guidepost to selected political interfaces that need careful thought and deliberation. It must be recognized that nursing matters are a fundamental component in the political milieu of any health care organization. It should come as no surprise that the prizes in democratic politics go to the active and the organized[14]. A key point with respect to nursing matters in a political environment has to do with the larger picture of societal norms and social dynamics. Any service organization must function within larger political arenas and, given consumer advocacy and federal regulation, is subject to various external social and political priorities. It is to nursing's advantage to be acquainted with those priorities and, at the least, function in other than opposition to those priorities. Further, nursing has a responsibility to work in an organized fashion to shape those priorities.

With respect to politics, nursing must overcome naivete, cynicism, ignorance, and political inertia to work more effectively in the health care environment. Nursing leaders have a responsibility to guide the less experienced through the web of political realities and give them a fundamental appreciation of political workings. It is hoped that the model presented in this article will contribute to that process. As noted by Leininger, the administrators of tomorrow will be handling a greater variety of political conflicts, power struggles, and competition for scarce resources than ever before in nursing[15]. Our modus operandi can no longer be reactionary. Rather, we must operate with both political knowledge and political skill.

References

1. Clark Kerr. "The Administration of Higher Education in an Era of Change and Conflict." First David D. Henry Lecture, University of Illinois, Urbana-Champaign, October 10-11, 1972.

2. Robert Dahl. *Who Governs* (New Haven, Conn.: Yale University Press, 1961).

3. Donald Schon, *Beyond the Stable State* (London: Temple Smith, 1971), p. 60.

4. Ben Lawrence and Allan Service, *Quantitative Approaches to Higher Education Management: Potential, Limits and Challenge,* ERIC/Higher Education Research Report no. 4, 1977, p. 60.

5. Aaron Wildavsky, *The Politics of the Budgetary Process,* 3rd ed: (Boston: Little, Brown, 1979), p. 11.

6. Jeffrey Pfeffer. *Power in Organizations* (Marshfield, Mass.: Pitman, 1981).

7. Aaron Wildavsky, 1979, p. 191.

8. Aaron Wildavsky, 1979, p. 191.

9. Aaron Wildavsky, 1979, p. 192.

10. Paul Diesing, *Reason in Society* (Urbana: University of Illinois Press, 1962), p. 228.

11. Donald Schon, 1971, pp. 31-60.

12. Herbert Simon, *Models of Man* (New York: Wiley, 1957).

13. R. Fulmer, *Management and Organization: An Introduction to Theory and Practice* (New York: Barnes and Noble, 1979) p. 53.

14. Aaron Wildavsky, 1979, p. 157.

15. Madeline Leininger, ''Political Nursing: Essentials for Health Service and Educational Systems of Tomorrow,'' *Nursing Administration Quarterly* 5(1):2, 1980.

Bibliography

Alinsky, Saul. *Rules for Radicals.* New York: Vintage Books, 1971.

Allen, R.F., and Kraft, C. "Discovering the Hospital Unconscious." *Hospital Forum* (January/February 1983): 12-19.

Anthony, William P. *Management Competencies and Incompetencies.* Reading, Massachusetts: Addison-Wesley, 1981.

Bolman, Lee G., and Deal, Terrence E. *Modern Approaches to Understanding and Managing Organizations.* San Francisco: Jossey-Bass, 1984.

Brown, L. David. *Managing Conflict at Organizational Interfaces.* Reading, Massachusetts: Addison-Wesley, 1983.

Cavanaugh, Denise E. "Gamesmanship: The Art of Strategizing." *Journal of Nursing Administration* 14(April 1985): 35-41.

Chater, Shirley Sears. "Creative Uses of Power" In Conway, Mary E., and Olga Andruskiw (eds). *Administrative Theory and Practice.* Norwalk, Connecticut: Appleton-Century-Crofts, 1983.

Cousteau, Voltaire. "How To Swim With Sharks: A Primer." *Perspectives in Biology and Medicine* 16(Summer 1978): 525-528. (Reprinted in *American Journal of Nursing* 81(October 1981).

Deal, Terrence E., and Kennedy, Allan A. *Corporate Cultures.* Reading, Massachusetts: Addison-Wesley, 1982.

Ehrat, Karen S. "A Model for Politically Astute Planning and Decision Making." *Journal of Nursing Administration* 13(September 1983): 29-35.

Georgopoulos, Basil G. "The Hospital as an Organization and Problem Solving System," in Magula, Mary (ed). *Understanding Organizations.* Wakefield, Massachusetts: Nursing Resources, 1982: 31.

Hill, Raymond E., and Collins-Eaglin, Jan. "Technical Professionals, Technical Managers and the Integration of Vocational Consciousness." *Human Resource Management,* 24(Summer 1985): 177-189.

Jackall, Robert. "Moral Mazes: Bureaucracy and Managerial Work." *Harvard Business Review* 61(September 1983): 122.

Jelinek, Mariann, Smircich, Linda, and Hirsh, Paul. "A Code of Many Colors." *Administrative Science Quarterly* 28 (1982): 331-338.

Kanter, Rosabeth Moss. "The Middle Manager As Innovator," *Harvard Business Review* 60(July/August 1982): 98.

Kanter, Rosabeth Moss. *The Change Masters.* New York: Simon and Schuster, 1983.

Kennedy, Marilyn Moats. *Powerbase: How To Build It/How To Keep It.* New York: Macmillan, 1984.

Kotter, John P. *Power in Management.* New York: AMACOM, 1979.

Ludeman, Ruth. "Fit or Misfit: A Comparison of Hospital and Nursing Managers' Perceptions of Their Roles and Their Organizations." In *Proceedings: Second Annual National Conference on Nursing Administration Research.* Richmond, Virginia: Virginia Commonwealth University, 1983: 219-240.

Machiavelli, Niccolo. *The Prince and the Discourses.* New York: Random House, 1950.

McMurray, Robert N. "Power and the Ambitious Executive." *Harvard Business Review* 52(November/December 1973): 69-74.

Pettigrew, Andrew. "On Studying Organizational Cultures." *Administrative Science Quarterly* 24(December 1979): 570-582.

Raelin, Joseph. "The Basis for the Professional's Resistance to Managerial Control." *Human Resource Management* 24 (Summer 1985): 147-173.

Randsepp, Eugene. "In Step With Power." *The Executive Female* (November/December 1984): 36-40.

Schein, Edgar H. *Organizational Culture and Leadership.* San Francisco: Jossey-Bass, 1985.

Schein, Virginia. "The Politics of Change." *Performance and Instruction Journal* 24(March 1985): 1-5.

Smircich, Linda. "Concepts of Culture and Organizational Analysis." *Administrative Science Quarterly* 28(September 1983): 339-358.

Tichy, Noel M. "Managing Organizational Transformations." *Human Resource Management* 22(Spring/Summer 1983): 45-60.

Ulrich, Wendy L. "HRM and Culture: History Ritual, and Myths." *Human Resource Management* 23(Summer 1984): 117-128.

Von Glinow, Mary Ann. "Reward Strategies for Attracting, Evaluating, and Retaining Professionals." *Human Resource Management* 24(Summer 1985): 191-206.

Wilkins, Alan L. "The Creation of Company Cultures: The Role of Stories and Human Resource Systems." *Human Resource Management* 23(Spring 1984): 41-60.

Wilkins, Alan L. "The Culture Audit: A Tool for Understanding Organizations." *Organizational Dynamics* (Autumn 1983): 24-38.

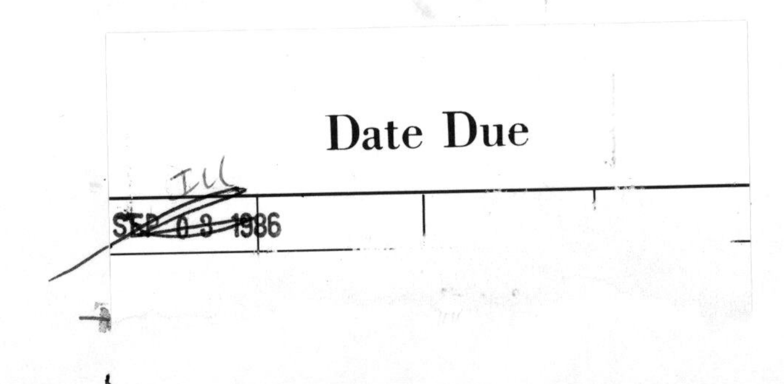